C000259054

The Chinese

Connection

'South of the Clouds'

Peggy Barnes

Abbie,

love Peggy

x x

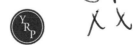

Yellow Rose Publishing Ltd

First published in United Kingdom in 2017 by

Peggy Barnes - YRP

A CIP catalogue record for this title is available from the British Library

ISBN 978-1-912320-04-2

Cover illustrations: Rufus Newell

Editor: Nicola Burrows

www.peggybarnes.co.uk

www.yellowrosepublishing.com

Disclaimer

I have tried to recreate events, locales and conversations from my memories of them. In order to maintain their anonymity in some instances I have changed some identifying characteristics.

Dedicated to:

My sons Chris and Mike,
and my lovely daughter Angie
who left this world in 2010.

"Seize the opportunity when it arises,
Once missed, it may be lost forever."

Feng Menglong
Chinese Writer and poet of the late Ming Dynasty
1574 - 1646

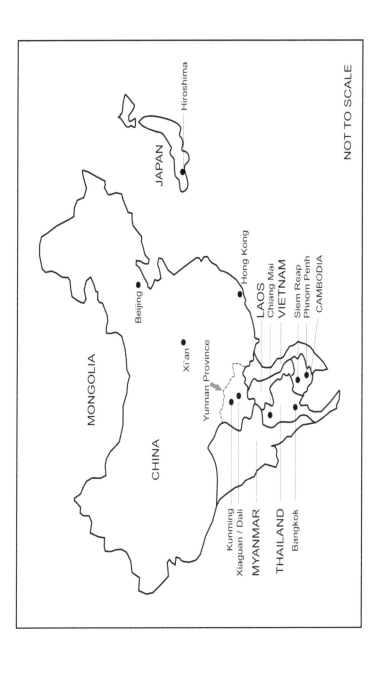

NOT TO SCALE

MONGOLIA

CHINA

JAPAN

Beijing

Hiroshima

Xi'an

Yunnan Province

Hong Kong

Kunming

Xiaguan / Dali

MYANMAR

LAOS

Chiang Mai

VIETNAM

THAILAND

Siem Reap

Phnom Penh

CAMBODIA

Bangkok

Foreword

The Golden Flower Girl

Peggy has kindly asked me to write a foreword to her account of her experience as a VSO volunteer in Dali in south west China in the last three years of the 20th century.

Our paths crossed after I lost my partner Barry to HIV in 1996, and I decided to create an English charity, Barry & Martin's Trust, to cooperate between the UK and China in HIV treatment and care.

Through my niece Nathalie, who had herself been a volunteer in China, I was told that Peggy had recently arrived in Dali and wanted expert help to train the local doctors and nurses in HIV care. We therefore sent a doctor and nurse from Chelsea & Westminster Hospital, Penny and Fiona, to join Peggy in an AIDS workshop in Dali.

This was early days in HIV care in China. Little was known, even in Beijing, and even less in a provincial town, far from the capital. Peggy was quick to recognise the need. Those early training sessions were met with some scepticism- but among the locals there was one outstanding doctor, Zhang Jianbuo, who was keen to take the project forward.

Most VSO volunteers were young graduates, and they were mostly sent in pairs to different parts of China (and to different parts of the world), and they were mainly training English teachers. Peggy was an exception, already a semi-retired nurse, and a grandmother, she was sent on her own to Dali- a challenge at any age.

Peggy arrived in the old town of Dali, in its spectacular setting between its mountains and its lake, at an interesting stage of the development of modern China. Peggy's book gives a glimpse of a country going through massive change. This work which an English nurse was able to achieve demonstrates the best spirit of volunteering, and a warmth which has continued to develop between Dali and England.

Dali has an extraordinary history. It was the home in particular of the Bai people, and a thousand years ago the kings of Dali ruled a vast empire, stretching from Chengdu to Hanoi, and they twice defeated the armies of the Tang emperors of China.

The connection of Dali with the United Kingdom goes back to 1886, when the London Inland Mission established a station there. This continued, on and off, until the Revolution in 1949. The missionaries who had built Dali's first hospital were not expelled until 1951.

To some extent, Peggy's arrival in Dali in 1997 enabled her to take up some of the historical links. The old work of the missionary hospital had not been forgotten, and some of the old staff were still living. Thus, the work of Peggy and of Dr Zhang Jianbuo was solidly based.

In the new century, after Peggy had left, the old hospital was restored by Barry & Martin's Trust and the local municipality, and we named it the Peggy Health Centre. It is regarded throughout China as a model of excellence in AIDS treatment and care, with the lowest mortality, the highest adherence, and the most regular attendance.

It is refreshing to record this continuity of Peggy's work, long after she has left Dali. It is no surprise that the local people named her the Golden Flower Girl.

Martin Gordon OBE,
Chairman of The Barry and Martin's Trust.

Prologue
November 2001

"Hello. Is that Peggy Barnes? This is Fiona from the British Embassy in Beijing. Are you on your own? I hope so because I've got some great news for you; you've been made a Member of the Order of the British Empire."

"I'm sorry Fiona. Would you repeat that please?" I asked in total disbelief.

"You've been given an MBE for your services to HIV and AIDS Awareness and Training in China. Congratulations from all at the Embassy."

I sat down, unable to believe my ears.

"Can I inform the Palace that you will accept the award?" she continued. "Yes," I whispered. "I'm suffering from shock right now, but I'll be delighted to accept the award. Thank you so much."

She went on to say that I should tell no one until the announcement appeared in the press at the end of December, and I know what followed was the longest six weeks of my life. I chose February 27th 2002 to attend the investiture at Buckingham Palace. After a great deal of thought and a little help from my friends, an embroidered Chinese jacket over a long red silk skirt seemed to be the right thing to wear for this auspicious occasion. I felt incredibly proud in the surreal surroundings as I made the journey through the grand entrance with my three children Angie, Chris and Mike by my side. They were the best friends I could have wished for and I was so lucky to have them with me. Once inside the Palace, the guests were escorted to the Grand Ballroom to await the investiture, while we recipients were shown to the Painting Room where a briefing took place in a relaxed and friendly atmosphere.

With the briefing fresh in my mind, I stood next to an equerry in the wings of the Grand Ballroom and waited for my name to be called. Music was being played by the band of the Irish Guards and I felt strangely calm.

"Margaret Barnes," the voice boomed out. Yes, it really was me being called by my proper name and, before I knew what was happening, I was actually in the Palace standing no more than a few inches from His Royal Highness, Prince Charles. He smiled and said, "You spent three years in a rural area in China, I believe. I'm sure you had some interesting experiences during that time."

"I certainly did," I replied, and so my story begins.

Chapter 1

I sat down and thought about my need to do something vastly different with my life. I'd spent almost all my working life as a State Registered Nurse in the British National Health Service, but my priorities began to change when I obtained a second divorce. What was I doing, and more importantly, where was I going? There were two choices open to me: I could remain in my job as a Specialist Nurse which I loved and found stimulating, or do something that might change my life forever. I spoke with many people hoping for guidance, but it didn't come. Days were spent in the public library researching different charities and agencies until eventually I found details about Voluntary Service Overseas (VSO), a charity which provided aid in developing countries. This organisation sent people rather than money and material things. The volunteers worked within the community in many of the world's poorest countries, sharing work, hopefully resulting in some long-lasting changes. This would present a real challenge, something I desperately needed. It would not only give me the opportunity to travel and live in another country, but enable me to share my skills and experience for the benefit of others.

I applied for consideration from VSO and was accepted. My family were delighted, but some of my friends thought I was plain crazy. They couldn't understand why I'd ever want a change in career, let alone to work in a foreign land so far away from everyone I knew and loved.

Early in 1996, I left the Health Service I'd known so well and started preparing for my new life. To broaden my experience, I joined a nursing agency which allowed me to work in a wide range of settings, enabling me to update my skills. Other days were spent on weekend courses with VSO in Birmingham. It was good to meet other like-minded individuals in a relaxed and friendly atmosphere and also learn about the workings of the organisation. The courses were excellent and went a long way towards preparing me for my 'new life.'

In June of that year I was ready for a placement. With mixed emotions, I visited the main office in London and considered offers of positions in a number of countries. I declined them all for various reasons when out of the blue a post in The People's Republic of China appeared. A two-year assignment in Xiaguan, a city in Yunnan Province in Southwest China, with a remit of improving the inpatient care in a new hospital affiliated to the nearby medical college was requested. I felt a shiver of excitement run through me and knew, without doubt, that this was where I was meant to go.

China, a Communist country with a population of some 1.2 billion, was huge and sat on the other side of the world. Much of the publicity I'd read in newspapers and magazines was restrained and negative, and there seemed to be a total lack of information regarding the poorest members of society.

Would I be confronted with hordes of men and women wearing shapeless blue Mao suits and matching blue cloth hats singing patriotic songs? I wanted to know more and decided to do some serious research on the area. I rummaged through books in the Public Library, but my newly acquired Lonely Planet Guide Book told me most. It said Yunnan Province was home not only to the ruling Han Chinese, but also to 26 colourful ethnic minority groups who had retained their costumes and interesting cultural practices. The Province itself was roughly the size of France, with a population of some 35 million. It bordered Myanmar or Burma, Laos and Vietnam. It was indeed a long way from Worcester, but I wasn't intimidated, accepted the offer, and guessed it wouldn't be easy move.

The journey to Xiaguan was going to be a long one. First to Beijing, then to Xi'an for a short in-service training period before heading off to Kunming, and finally a long trip by road to the city of Xiaguan. Some financial backup would be essential. Although I would receive a small monthly salary, emergencies could always happen so I decided to take some cash and my bank cards. With my security assured, I was ready to go.

Chapter 2

After farewell hugs and kisses to my family and dear friend Margaret, I stood alone in the departure terminal at Heathrow Airport. My legs felt like jelly. What on earth had I done? I was in a daze and felt as if I was on another planet as I watched my rucksack disappear on the conveyor belt bound for Beijing. Was I going mad? Four hours earlier I had been sitting on my bed surrounded by everything VSO had advised me to take: clothes and footwear for the differing seasons plus toilet rolls and tissues, although how I was to make these last for two years I didn't know. There were books, including The Royal Marsden Manual of Clinical Nursing, my precious address book, a CD player and a few carefully selected discs by Queen, Phil Collins and Eric Clapton. A short-wave radio was painstakingly tucked in with make-up and toiletries and somehow, I managed to cram everything into my bag.

The decision to do something dramatic had been easy to make a year ago. With all the training I'd received from VSO I thought I was thoroughly prepared, but now I felt sick and was unsure. Confronted with reality I wanted to back out on this day, February 12th 1997, but my pride wouldn't allow me. This was the Chinese year of the Ox, a year for leaders who naturally inspire confidence in others, or so I'd been told. I'd been born in the year of the Pig, whose people are home lovers. This emphasised my dilemma. Should I go? I tried to look confident, but deep down felt I would fail miserably.

The adrenaline began to flow as I searched the departure terminal for my travelling companions, the thirty English teachers I'd been told to join. I had briefly met two of them, Norma and Jean, at one of the VSO courses in Birmingham a few months before, but where were they now? And what did the rest of the group look like? I didn't have to wait too long as we had a block booking on a Jumbo. Almost before we settled into our seats we were introducing ourselves and I decided we were a somewhat motley collection of individuals of mixed ages with many things in common. Some had recently completed university studies while others, like me, were approaching retirement. We were an untidy, noisy group which gelled immediately. We tried to settle for the night flight to Beijing, but for most there was little sleep. We were full of excitement at the start of an adventure and too busy getting to know each other during the nine and a half hours flying time. The journey took us over Europe and Russia in complete darkness. When daylight broke, I looked out over the vast Gobi Desert.

I wondered what lay ahead. There was nothing to be seen through the window but snow, snow and more snow. Occasionally straight black lines came into view. They seemed to go on forever and broke up the huge expanses of white. They could have been railway tracks, but I never did find out.

Eventually the whiteness gave way to grey, and at dawn we landed at Beijing Airport.

"Hi. Welcome to Beijing. We are your VSO programme officers. When you've collected your luggage, come over here please," yelled Sean, one of the three in-country staff who had come to meet us. "We won't waste any time. The coaches are outside and there will be refreshments for you at the hotel."

I knew there were programme officers based in the capital. They were VSO staff and each one had been allocated an area in China. Part of their role was to organise the orientation programme, which included basic language training. They were also there to oversee the individual projects and provide support to each volunteer.

The bus journey to the city took an hour on a dual carriageway. Tall leafless trees, festooned with rags, bits of paper and pink plastic bags, lined the highway and everything looked dreary and dull. Clumps of grey buildings looked as if they had been erected in boring rectangular grids. There was no colour except for the odd red flag that fluttered in the breeze. Even the fields were grey-brown, no doubt from the effects of a harsh winter. All very different from pictures I'd seen in the glossy travel brochures promising sunshine and bright colours

Our hotel on the outskirts of the city looked pretty grim from the outside. It was even more depressing on the inside, with a dreary and poorly lit reception area manned by an unsmiling girl. For certain it would never have won any awards for its hospitality or welcoming ambience. My room had all the essentials and the bed was clean and fresh, but as I showered in the mildew-covered unit I was relieved to know we would only be there one night. Nevertheless, I did feel better after a clean-up and a change of clothing, and returned to the reception area in a light-hearted mood to meet the others. There was only a day and a half in the city before we were to set off for our in-service training in Xi'an, a city in Shaanxi Province some distance away. Several of us sat round a large table, and as we drank green tea and nibbled at some dubious looking cake, Norma, Jean and I made a snap decision to visit the famous Tiananmen Square.

Warily, we ventured outside for our first look at Beijing. The pollution hit our throats and made us cough and splutter. It was bitterly cold. The traffic was insane. Men were hanging around in small groups and most were hawking, coughing and spitting. An old man, wobbling along on a bike with a gas cylinder tied either side of the crossbar, almost bowled me over on my first attempt to step into the road. He obviously couldn't stop and I had looked the wrong way. During the last year I had read a lot about China and one fact among the many I'd learned was the vast quantity of almost everything, including people. Can you imagine a city with eleven million people and nine million bikes all on the move? There were buses, cars, motorcycles, bicycles, rickshaws, pedestrians and peasants with laden bamboo poles balanced on their shoulders. Everyone seemed to be trying to navigate the crowded thoroughfares at the same time.

A hailed taxi whisked the three of us to the Square, a journey that proved a nightmare with a driver who behaved as if he was on a race track. We were on the brink of hysteria when we reached our destination and were more than happy to get our feet back on terra firma.

Tiananmen Square is the largest of its type in the world. I had read about it and knew something of its history. However, the first time I stood in the heart of it, I was stunned by its vastness. The level area was covered in grey paving slabs broken only by large buildings shrouded in smog.

My guidebook said Chairman Mao had created this Square in 1949 and it was here, during the Cultural Revolution, that he reviewed parades of tens of thousands of people.

"My God, this place is enormous. I feel so small and insignificant now I'm actually standing here. Do you feel the same?" I asked my friends. They both nodded.

"I can't see any trees or grass. The whole place feels empty, grey and eerie which is strange because there are hundreds of people about. And look at all those beautiful kites. I've never seen so many in the air at the same time," Jean said as we gazed upwards.

The paper frames looked like fragile birds as they swooped and pirouetted, with their tails fluttering and rustling as they were flown higher and higher. Their simple beauty captivated us. Of course, it wasn't long before these kite flyers were trying to sell them to us, along with postcards and other memorabilia.

There was real excitement in Norma's voice as she touched my arm. "That must be Chairman Mao Zedong's tomb over there," she said.

Neither of us had ever seen a Mausoleum before and the building was massive. Somehow just looking at it made me feel that the power this man had once held over the entire population was still present. Sadly, a barrier was in position and we couldn't go inside. Next to Chairman Mao's resting place stood the Monument to the Peoples' Heroes. It had been completed in 1958 and important historical events were carved on the surface in Chinese characters, which we couldn't understand. This tall impressive building dwarfed us as we gazed skyward in awe. Nearby, we saw the Great Hall of the People. It seemed to be covered in a mass of red flags in perfectly straight lines. After climbing the steps to the entrance we found the doors tightly closed, obviously not a place for tourists on that day.

We joined countless Chinese to watch as the National Flag was lowered at sunset by a troop from The People's Liberation Army, resplendent in their uniforms. This act of patriotism was striking and again we reflected on the discipline of a nation still obviously influenced by their late leader Mao Zedong.

In the distance we could see the Tiananmen, or Heavenly Peace Gate, with the huge portrait of Chairman Mao sometimes known as the Great Helmsman. He appeared to be scanning the crowds, including us, as we set out to cross the road towards it, via a subway. This underground walkway was crowded with beggars. Some were lying on the ground, obviously thin and ill. Others elbowed their way to the front to beg. We hastily transferred our small backpacks to our chests and wrapped our arms around them to deter pickpockets. Judging by the way other people clutched their bags it was a sound move.

We emerged from the darkness in front of the huge portrait. We had to have a reminder of this moment and posed, along with some Chinese, to have our photos taken by a friendly guard before making our way through the Gate, towards The Forbidden City.

To get there we had to pass what seemed like dozens of stalls selling piles and piles of kites, tacky curios and 'I've been to Beijing' T-shirts. These stall holders had a different attitude to that of the kite sellers in the Square; they seemed totally disinterested. Maybe they were employed by the government and paid a wage, or perhaps it was the end of the day for them.

A large notice informed us the last tickets to gain entry to the Forbidden City were sold to the public at half past three. We were too late to enter. Our guidebooks said this huge collection of red, high-walled, well-preserved buildings behind the Gate had not only been the seat of government but also the playground of the Ming and Qing Dynasties for the last five hundred years. We had to be content with a walk around the perimeter. We were both excited and tired and, as the cold had intensified, we hailed another taxi and endured another hellish ride back to our hotel.

After a quick tidy up, we met the other volunteers for a meal. The memories of it will remain with me forever. Most of it was like nothing I'd ever encountered. One dish resembled a stew with gristly meat and dollops of fat floating on the top. In a bowl next to it, shredded cabbage sat in the water it had been boiled in. There was a huge basin of rice, a large plate of greasy chips and a bowl of tofu swimming in something unmentionable. I normally have a go at anything, but the texture of warm lumps of tasteless, slimy tofu made me feel sick. I began to realise how versatile the Chinese were in adapting their cuisine to the taste of so many cultures worldwide. But today, my introduction to real Chinese food was one I didn't want to repeat in a hurry. The hunger pangs were making my stomach rumble, and I wasn't alone.

"Hey," said John, who was sitting next to me, "there's a MacDonald's over there. It's sure to be OK and at least we'll know what we're eating, I hope. Who's coming with me?"

It wasn't long before most of our group made our way to the well-known fast food restaurant, guided by the familiar golden arches. The burgers and fries went down well, as did the beer in a nearby drinking house. At the end of the evening most of us felt a lot more receptive to whatever the future held for us.

The following morning, we were taken to the British Embassy and introduced to the Consul and his wife. This charming couple made us most welcome and, after registration, treated us to numerous cups of tea, dainty sandwiches and sponge cakes. They gave us several books and articles on

Britain, which would undoubtedly be useful at some stage within our placements.

Next it was off by coach to see the Great Wall. Again, we had to run the gauntlet of shops and stalls that surrounded the entrance. It was the same tacky produce we'd seen on the Square and at the entrance to the Forbidden City, only this time the T-shirts boasted 'I've been to the Great Wall'. Once more the sellers seemed to be totally disinterested in either our money or us. I did get some action though, when I fell for a Chinese army-style fur hat with lovely big, floppy earmuffs, and received my first lesson in haggling. I thought I'd got a great deal when I offered half the asking price. When I saw the grin on the stallholder's face, I wasn't quite so sure.

Our cameras clicked non-stop as we took our first steps on the Wall. I was thrilled to walk a little way along this amazing structure. In perfect English, our Chinese guide told us this part of the Wall was constructed over many centuries to repel marauding bandits, in particular the Manchurians and the Mongols. My mind began to run riot as I imagined hundreds of desperados attempting to clamber over this immense two thousand five-hundred-year-old fortification. It was obvious they'd never succeed; the structure was daunting. What we could see of the Wall seemed to go on forever, like a long white snake weaving its way through valleys, up hillsides and over mountains.

There were so many Beijing treasures, such as the Mausoleum, the Great Hall of the People, the Old Summer

Palace, the Forbidden City and Tiantan Park and countless others. We hadn't a hope to see any of these on this visit but we felt optimistic that a further opportunity would arise sometime in the future. We packed that evening in readiness for our flight to Xi'an the following day.

Chapter 3

It was approaching dusk as we circled above the mushroom cloud of pollution over Xi'an and by the time we reached our destination it was pitch dark. Our bus drew to a halt within walking distance of the Cuiyan Guest House, part of the North-West University where our induction course was to take place. Judging by what I could see it looked to be a typical student accommodation block, and this was to be our home for the next two and a half weeks.

As I got off the coach, the pavement gave way and I almost disappeared down a hole. I froze with horror, but the sound of a snap in my right foot brought me to my senses. Oh my god what had I done. It was not so much the pain I was concerned with at that moment, it was the sudden arrival of a colleague who landed on top of me, not realising my predicament. After what seemed like an eternity the coach moved forward a little to allow us to struggle out. With help from the rest of the group I recovered my possessions and was able to limp the hundred metres or so to the guesthouse. In reception I watched my foot swell at an alarming rate. Packs of ice cubes and painkilling tablets dulled the persistent ache for a short while, as did a couple of bottles of beer, but in the end I knew I'd have to grin and bear it. I struggled to my room, feeling depressed and useless.

That night seemed endless. The initial soothing effect of tablets had vanished and constant throbbing combined with the racket of nocturnal building construction ensured the most I could achieve that night was fitful dozing. The builders were working on the adjacent block and it seemed there were dozens of them laying bricks and mixing concrete. Their voices rose above the clatter of their tools, while dust billowed above the new concrete like belching power stations. When daylight broke I was exhausted but relieved as I would be able to get some help. After dressing I hopped to meet a programme officer. I knew I had to see a doctor and together we went by taxi to the Xi'an Number One Peoples' Hospital. I was about to get an early introduction to the Chinese Health System.

At six-thirty in the morning the city was alive with cars, trucks, bikes, pedestrians, along with horses and carts. They jostled for position on the road as dozens of men and women prepared food in woks with their cooking facilities sitting precariously on tables and trolleys that littered the rough pavements. Smoke and flames filled the air as people clutched bowls and chopsticks, eating their breakfasts as they gossiped. The thought crossed my mind that this street food might taste a great deal better than the stuff on offer at the Guesthouse. But we couldn't stop. My foot had to take priority.

At the hospital we were directed to the Foreigners' Section for registration and that's when I discovered there were no wheelchairs. My foot throbbed and my heart sank. Suppressing a smile at the picture conjured in my mind's eye, I declined the receiving officer's offer to carry me 'piggy back' style. I was at least twice her size. So, with gritted teeth, the hopping started all over again. The hospital was an extremely large, dreary grey concrete building with the Emergency Unit at the far end. I prayed that my left leg would keep me upright, and with grim determination succeeded in reaching the correct department.

Not only was this my first visit to a Chinese hospital, it was the first time I'd been in close contact with Chinese people. When we arrived at the Emergency Department I leaned against the wall and took a good look around. There were sick people and their companions everywhere, some being carried on the backs of relatives and others being helped in a more conventional manner. Dead bodies with small white cloths covering their faces occupied the only trolleys I could see. There was a buzz of constant chatter and the odd hawk, cough and spit. This was a far cry from the Accident and Emergency Units I was familiar within our British Health Service.

I joined the queue to see the doctor, who was working alone, and resigned myself to a long wait. There was no privacy whatsoever; not a curtain or screen in sight. People were being stripped and examined while scores of others looked on, apparently accepting the situation. Relatives were caring for their loved ones and managing as best they could. Eventually, my turn came and a gap was made through the crowd so I could hop to an examination couch. I concealed my revulsion at the sight of a dirty white sheet that covered it, reasoning it was best ignored as the doctor did a quick assessment.

"Bone broken," he said and pointed to the X-ray department. This unit was nearby and a fracture in a metatarsal just below my ankle was confirmed by a large machine which was slowly lowered from the ceiling. It sounded like a small helicopter landing beside me.

The next trip was to the Plaster Room, which unfortunately was upstairs. I took a deep breath and was grateful that there were banisters. It didn't take me long to realise I couldn't use them and had to slowly zigzag my way upward between blobs of green, sloppy sputum. Strategically placed spittoons had been totally missed or ignored, and this was in a hospital.

I recalled my placement remit and wondered with dismay if things were the same in every hospital. Little wonder the purpose of my visit was education! However this was not the time to be concerned for the future. I had to accept the present situation. Three men in white uniforms awaited my arrival. At last I could sit and take in my predicament. I watched as a tape measure was produced and my leg measured. One technician took a new Plaster of Paris bandage out of its wrapper and knelt on the dirty floor. With a cloth he cleared some of the dust, sputum and cigarette butts before he unrolled the dressing and calculated the required length necessary on the same surface. The only fairly clean thing I could see was the bowl of water that the bandage was soaked in before it was wound around my leg. I was so relieved not to have any broken skin because the risk of infection must have been high. The technician told me the Plaster of Paris bandage would take about three weeks to dry, but I wasn't surprised. I could see it was a very old type. The important thing was to get my ankle healed and I'd accepted the differences in the treatment between East and West. My VSO colleague paid up front, but the costs of my entire treatment would be met by the VSO medical insurance.

Finally, four hours after registration, my treatment was complete and I headed back to the university. My left leg ached from hopping. The toes on my right foot were swollen and blue but my fractured metatarsal was safely encapsulated in a wet and cold plaster bandage. It would have to stay like that for six weeks.

The next few days were not good. At first I had no crutches and had to continue hopping. I was frustrated and wept frequently. My new friends waited on me at mealtimes and generally looked after me but I missed great chunks of the induction course simply because I couldn't get upstairs. I did manage a few sessions in the Chinese language, Mandarin, which in due course became more than useful. Most evenings were spent with a group of fellow volunteers keeping me company in my room. These new friends were great and kept me amused with tales of the day's events as we supped bottles of beer.

During the weekend, a trip was arranged to the Terracotta Warriors. I really wanted to go but couldn't imagine how I would manage. Once more my fellow volunteers stepped in and shoulder-carried me around the three vaults. What a day! What an amazing sight – a collection of underground rooms containing thousands of life-sized terracotta warriors and their horses, all facing east. There was row upon row of them. Some local peasants discovered them in 1974 near the Tomb of Qin Shihuang. Since then many more have been discovered.

The next few evenings at the hostel were spent with me repaying my gallant VSO friends with beer and massaging their shoulders. To everyone's relief, a pair of elbow crutches eventually arrived from the British Embassy in Beijing. At last I was mobile, albeit a bit wobbly.

With the completion of the induction course we had to say goodbye to each other and set off for our respective schools, colleges and in my case, a hospital. We were going to many different parts of the country. I was one of the few flying to my placement. Most of my colleagues were travelling by train. The support offered by the VSO staff in Xi'an was fine and the friendly atmosphere in the hostel was welcome. The beer kept most of us in good spirits and in such close quarters we got to know each other well. Now we had to go, but knowing that some of us would probably meet up during the summer vacation and definitely in November at the Annual Conference, the parting was not too traumatic.

Chapter 4

A taxi arrived to take me to the airport for my flight to Kunming, the first leg of my journey to Xiaguan.

The driver smiled and said "No English" as he helped me into his car.

I was silent as we sped along the highway and took little comfort from the car driver's repeated mutterings of 'no problem, no problem'. Once at the airport he leapt out of the car and disappeared from view for a couple of minutes before returning with an even bigger smile and a wheelchair. I was grateful to be wheeled into the departures area, where we stopped briefly at the check-in counter and my luggage was whisked away. A boarding card was thrust into my hand and the next thing I knew I was in the departure lounge where I thanked the driver and waved him goodbye.

I sat patiently only to discover that the flight was delayed for three hours. Thus, the waiting began and another lesson in tolerance was made worse by my urgent need for a visit to the toilet. I was glad to have a book to read to keep myself occupied. Eventually boarding commenced and all other passengers headed towards the designated channel whilst I was alone and deserted. In the end four uniformed men appeared and, without a word, escorted me down the tunnel. Suddenly the passageway was no more and, as we turned left, I was hoisted up and airborne with a man at each corner of my wheelchair. Ahead of me was a set of steep steps and my eyes were shut tight as we descended. I was flooded with relief when we reached tarmac and opted to hobble up the steps to board my plane.

It was a good flight to Kunming. I had been allocated two seats in the front and was able to negotiate the toilet. The three-hour flight was trouble free and as I had been assured I would be met on my arrival, I relaxed and enjoyed the scenery below. Sure enough, two Chinese women were waiting as I came through the gate in my wheel chair and I breathed a sigh of relief.

"Hi," said a smiling face, "I'm Zhang Rumei, your interpreter. This is Miss Li, head nurse of the new hospital. As she speaks no English I'll be doing the talking. Mr Chan, our driver, has gone to fetch the car. He'll be here soon and we'll get you to your hotel for the night. Please call me Rumei; I'll be working with you as your interpreter and I know we'll soon get to know each other well."

Rumei was tall, slim and pretty. Her dark eyes sparkled and her black hair was tied in a ponytail. She looked immaculate in a maroon trouser suit. Miss Li, who was not quite as tall, had short black hair. She was wearing a black trouser suit. Her face was expressionless as she extended her hand in welcome. A smiling Mr Chan helped us into the car and

I was taken for a one-night stay at the Camellia Hotel in East Dong Feng Road in the heart of the city.

That evening, Rumei and Miss Li took me to meet three people who worked in the city with three different Non-Governmental Organisations, or NGO's.

"Hi. We're glad to meet you, Peggy, and welcome to Kunming. I'm Kate with Save the Children Organisation. This is Audrey, from Yunnan/Australian Red Cross, and this is another Peggy, who's with Medecins Sans Frontieres. We are all based here in the city and are linked by our interest and education in the HIV and AIDS field. You're a Registered nurse I believe, and I think you already know Chinese hospitals are a little bit different from ours," she said as she turned her eyes towards my plastered leg.

Over a coffee we relaxed and got to know each other. It was good to realise that I had fairly close neighbours who were like-minded and relaxed. Ultimately these three people were to become not only good friends, but also reliable sources of information as my role evolved.

Kunming, known as Spring City, is the capital of Yunnan Province. In the dim evening light I could see azaleas, camellias and magnolias in bloom along the roadside. Rows of shops with bright lights blazing stood behind them and in the background were well-lit blocks of tall grey apartment buildings. As I was drifting off to sleep in my hotel bed I felt I'd had a pleasant, albeit brief, introduction to the city and it felt good.

At seven o'clock in the morning Rumei, Ms Li, Mr Chan the driver, and I sat at a small table outside a café to have a breakfast of noodle soup. I'd never used chopsticks before and found the spicy food and slippery noodles a major problem. The chillies made my eyes water and tears streamed down my face. My nose ran and I felt a real mess. I was more than a bit embarrassed when I realised a crowd had gathered to watch my struggle, so I gave up and left the meal unfinished. Looking up, I was thankful that Mr Chan had brought the car. He was ready to leave so I quickly climbed into the back seat with Rumei, and settled down to have a good look at the local life.

The whole city seemed to be on the move. There were peddlers laden with produce in buckets hanging from bamboo shoulder poles, shoppers with swollen bags, mammoth bus queues and countless buses bulging with standing commuters. I saw what seemed like hundreds of bikes, burdened with everything from animal carcasses and cabbages to small children, homemade brooms and textiles. I was silent as I absorbed the scenes continually unfolding before me as we drove through the capital towards the dual carriageway. As the city disappeared behind me I caught a glimpse of Lake Dian with the sun sparkling on the waters. Kunming was a riot of colour and noise. I loved the action and looked forward to the day when I could return to spend time wandering around at my leisure. I'm keen on shopping and couldn't find any reason to change just because I was in a foreign country!

The sun streamed through tall trees as we headed towards Xiaguan. Their trunks were painted white, presumably to prevent insect or beetle infestation. They looked like a column of orderly soldiers bordering each side of the road to maintain a steady flow of traffic. Mountain ranges and neatly cultivated valleys surrounded us. Periodically, small villages of mud walled houses with thatched roofs appeared. The eaves, with little house gods made of straw standing on each corner, swept up towards the heavens and made a picturesque sight. These family homes were joined by a series of tamped-mud paths. I was fascinated as I watched the hundreds of peasants, each one working his small area with a hoe, and not one tractor in sight. My companions thought that I was a little strange as I gazed non-stop out of the window. They didn't realise everything I saw was so different from the Worcestershire countryside I'd left behind such a short time ago. I knew this was probably an extremely poor part of China, but had not yet enough experience for comparison.

Rumei had told me that a new road from Kunming to Xiaguan was being built because the old road passed through all the towns and villages was narrow and a new dual carriageway would shorten the four hundred kilometre journey considerably. The promised road works were well underway. We stopped and started many times as we bumped our way over and around huge potholes. There were long queues of traffic and we took endless detours on dirt roads with sheer drops. There were no crash barriers as we went up and over mountains and I didn't like to think of the consequences if our driver made a wrong move.

Miss Li remained quiet and a weird tension had crept into the atmosphere. I wondered if I had inadvertently breached some protocol. The silences were uncomfortable and made me feel uneasy. This was going to be a long journey. We paused at the roadside in a traffic hold up and our driver decided that we had enough time to stretch our legs. I struggled from the car and sat on a rock ledge, glad to be away from the tense atmosphere. I lit a cigarette and offered one to Mr Chan when he sat by my side. We couldn't chat to one another, but somehow the smoking of a cigarette bonded us, and for the rest of the journey I sat next to him in the front passenger seat of the car. This was a big break, I felt much more comfortable and settled back to enjoy the beauty of the countryside despite the endless road works.

The next stop was at a small roadside café for food and a comfort stop. It wasn't long before I made my way to the lavatory, only to be confronted with my first squat latrine. I stood and looked at the two small holes strategically placed in the concrete floor. The place was filthy. It was awash with dirty water and great lumps of soiled toilet paper and much more. So much for the advice on bringing toilet rolls to the country that had probably invented them. I quickly decided this was no place for me with a plastered foot, so muttered a little prayer, and resolved to refrain from all fluids until we arrived in Xiaguan. On this occasion, and on many others over the next three years, I think I was extremely lucky to be spared what must have been the stench of the many latrines I was to encounter. I have no sense of smell whatsoever, the result of head injuries sustained in a road traffic accident when I was eighteen. However, I am also aware that I now live a life starkly bereft of what must be, without doubt, the most evocative of the five senses we normally possess.

After fifteen hours of rough roads, traffic jams, exhaust fumes and mountain drops, we reached the new Affiliated Hospital in Xiaguan. The relief of having finally arrived was mingled with exhaustion and a strange feeling of elation as I embarked upon this new chapter in my life.

Chapter 5

My employers were standing in a row at the hospital gate to greet me. With Rumei, my interpreter, by my side I was immediately introduced to two Chinese men, Yousheng Shu whose English name was David and Hongqi Yang known as Charles, the officers from the Foreign Affairs Department at the nearby medical college. They both spoke perfect English and made me feel welcome. Introductions to the rest of the group followed and my head was in a whirl. My head nurse friend, Miss Li, totally ignored me and I began to feel more than a little anxious again. I was hoping for a kindred spirit to help improve nursing standards, whatever they were. I wondered if her coolness was due to cultural misunderstanding. Perhaps I would find out.

After endless speeches, I was invited to say my first few words, when I told them how happy I was to be in Xiaguan and how much I looked forward to seeing their new hospital. Inwardly I wondered if I would remember all these faces and names. Secretly I was dying to ask for a toilet but the time never seemed right, so I had to put my greatest need to the back of my mind. I tried to keep it occupied as we headed for a large restaurant for the promised banquet with me as the honoured guest, and more speeches.

How I wished I had known something about the Chinese eating ritual. Who should sit down first – the host or me? Eventually I gave up and just sat down, hoping to avoid a diplomatic incident.

At each setting there was a bowl, a small dish of hot chilli dip and chopsticks. Everyone had a bottle of Dali beer and quite suddenly there was a great clinking of glasses and a shout of 'gan bei,' or bottoms up. The host downed his beer in one gulp and everyone followed suit. The men seemed to swallow air, but this was obviously fine, it just assisted with the belches that followed and nobody took any notice. More bottles of beer were opened and our glasses were immediately refilled by a couple of attentive waitresses. Opened bottles were not to be wasted. I had to slowly sip mine or be in serious trouble with my full bladder.

Local dishes, and there were many, kept on coming. In the centre of the round table a large fish was sitting on a special plate. Its dead eyes never seemed to leave me all evening. It stared at me from behind the pot of boiled black-skinned chicken and plates of crabs, prawns, pork and steamed pig cheek, daring me to try everything.

I guessed all the dishes were cooked to Chinese perfection. The table was well laid out and the red-hot chilli dip certainly flavoured the food. Mao-tai, a fiery sorghum spirit, or Chinese whisky, so they said, was drunk after all the toasts. This happened when the beer was finished. In my tired state it seemed to happen every five minutes or so. It was always a

'Gan bei' or 'Cheers' affair and the first time I downed the small glass of the stuff I thought my tonsils had been ripped off and it didn't taste much like any whisky I'd ever known. Nonetheless, I recovered well and managed quite a few more that evening. There were numerous ashtrays scattered at intervals and I soon discovered that not only was it possible, but also quite acceptable, to smoke and eat at the same time and I was only too willing to follow suit. It seemed to be usual thing to speak with a mouthful as well, and any food my hosts didn't like they simply spat on to the floor which was quickly littered with tissues, bones and more. The use of toothpicks appeared to be compulsory, but had to be done discreetly with a hand over the mouth.

I watched in bewilderment as whole crabs were munched complete with claws. Then entire prawns, heads, legs and all disappeared together with hard-boiled eggs complete with shells. I tried not to stare as I busied myself with an unidentifiable piece of chicken, full of bone splinters. I wasn't really hungry. Anyway, how much food did they expect me to eat? And what about all the hungry people I had been told about?

During the course of the evening not one person mentioned the fact that the hospital hadn't been completed, even though several individuals made long presentations about the project. I was to discover the partly built institution the following day. I had received my first lesson in not 'losing face'.

I was relieved, quite literally, when the festivities finally ended and I was taken to my third-floor apartment. I was left to my western-style toilet, my thoughts and myself.

Chapter 6

I felt edgy as I explored my new flat. It was within the grounds of the hospital, which was affiliated to the Dali Medical College a few kilometres away. I remembered having been told that everyone who worked in the unit also lived within the compound, known as a 'danwei'. It was completely fenced off and uniformed guards stood at the gates to protect it from the public. To me this seemed strange, but everything was different here and I would doubtless get used to it.

The basic kitchen comprised of a small single electric hob, a sink unit, a twin tub washing machine, a huge Chinese thermos flask, a fridge and two wooden storage cupboards. One contained a few plates, bowls, cups and chopsticks while the other housed a wok. The bathroom was off the kitchen and, to my great relief, consisted of a western toilet, a hand-washbasin and a bath with a shower unit fixed to the wall. The living room had a hard, uncomfortable three-piece suite, similar to those thrown on the tip back home, a television set and a small table. A dining room, with a huge table and six chairs, opened onto an empty balcony. My bedroom had bright yellow curtains at the window and a double bed was against a wall. The bottom sheet, which had the appearance of a huge towel, was covered with a flock duvet. A shiny red, yellow and orange cover was spread over the bedding and satin pillow slips with huge fluffy, gaudy flowers sewn onto them were placed in the centre. A built-in wardrobe and a dressing table with an ornate mirror stood nearby. None of the bulbs had shades and the naked lights shone harshly on the unforgiving grey concrete floor, casting mysterious shadows. There were few home comforts but I guessed if nothing else, the surface would be easy to clean.

With my plastered leg dangling over the side of the bath I managed to have a shower and eventually snuggled into my bed amidst the flowers. I smiled. The garish, glittery materials reminded me of the interior of a gypsy caravan I once visited in the wilds of Worcestershire during my district nursing days many years ago. I was tired but happy and slept well.

Chapter 7

The following morning, I could hardly believe my eyes as I looked out of my windows. To my right, the stunning peaks of the Cangshan Mountains cast long brown and green shadows as dawn broke. To my left four large junks were sailing on Erhai Lake and the waters were rippling soft colours in their wake. Unfortunately, the immediate vicinity wasn't so beautiful. There were numerous untidy piles of builders' rubbish from unfinished blocks of flats and other buildings and a couple of acres of barren, scrubby land. The large, white tiled construction standing to my right was presumably the new hospital. Hardly anyone was about. It was like a ghost town. What had I come to?

Rumei, my interpreter, was first to arrive with some noodles and vegetables for my breakfast. She was unhurried as step-by-step she showed me how to cook these fresh items in a wok and the end result was delicious. This lovely girl had been shopping and bought me provisions for the day. I was grateful, and, although I didn't recognise all the ingredients, I was prepared to have a go for my evening meal. Mid-morning four white-coated men arrived, each showing great interest in my plastered leg.

"The doctors don't seem to be too happy with the treatment you had in Xi'an and they want to look at your ankle." said Rumei.

My heart sank, my foot was comfortable, but I was well aware that one consultant didn't always agree with another so I consented to another X-ray, which did indeed reveal a problem. One of the doctors, Yang Kaishun, spoke a little English and I was soon to understand that my metatarsal had to be reset. Plaster of Paris was rarely used in this part of the world because of the cost, and most broken bones were simply set and splinted with willow or bamboo splints, and left to heal with time. My fracture treatment was new for some of my visitors and there was great interest. I was taken to a local clinic where a plaster saw was eventually found, and the work began. The damned stuff had taken nearly three weeks to dry, and being rock hard it needed a sharp knife and brute strength to remove it as the saw was more than slightly blunt. Finally, my foot was freed and I could see the protruding bone poking through under the skin. None of the medical team could really tell me what was about to happen, but I knew. Without more ado, Yang Kaishun looked me straight in the eye, muttered the word pain, and pressed the bone into the right position. I just held my breath and nearly squeezed the arm off the poor long-suffering Rumei.

A new cast was applied, but I was back to square one with wet, soggy plaster for three weeks then another month to wait before it was removed. I was more than a little fed up. The doctor gave me painkillers and Chinese medicines in little folded paper parcels and took me home.

I was frustrated and wept tears of anger. The new hospital was not functioning, there were few staff on site, and my foot was painful. One thing for sure, I would have plenty of time to prepare my teaching sessions and try to understand the head nurse. I suppose I could have returned to the UK, but my determination didn't allow me to consider that option. I had come to do a job, face a new challenge and would not be defeated.

A few days later Rumei arranged to take me out for a meal. I was not only to meet some of her colleagues from the Medical College, but also her five-year-old daughter. Little Xinran was the image of her mother with her black hair and sallow skin. She was a delightful little soul, and loved the applause she received after singing and dancing to her favourite songs. The six English teachers taught a variety of subjects and without exception spoke good English. Two had visited Scotland on an exchange basis and one had enjoyed a two-week holiday in Yorkshire with a previous VSO teacher. They all made me feel welcome without being patronising and wanted to learn more about ordinary life in Great Britain. It was a welcome feeling to have made new friends. They loved the photos of my friends and family I had put together in an album before I'd left home. The blond hair and blue eyes most of my grand-children provided great interest.

Rumei was an English teacher at the medical college and been allocated to me for the term. She took care of me until I was mobile, doing all my shopping and household tasks. Every day she came and we chatted about her home life and family. She gave me cooking lessons and I soon became an expert with a wok and knew, even then, I couldn't have managed without her in those early days. Walking round the flat was difficult enough, and going to the shops to buy food was impossible. One day she organised a taxi to take me to her parents' home. The couple were charming and remained my friends throughout the whole of my stay in China. They lived near the hospital and her father, a real gentleman, was a retired English teacher who enjoyed practising his language skills. Later I learned he had suffered at the hands of his students during 'struggle sessions' at some stage during the Cultural Revolution which occurred between 1966 and 1976.

This was a terrifying period in Chinese history when Mao Zedong tried to rid the country of the 'Four Olds', old customs, old culture, old habits and old thoughts. He closed all schools, most educational establishments and ordered the students to join the Red Guards Unit, which in turn tracked down teachers and intellectuals.

There was widespread book burning and a mass relocation of people from the cities to the countryside. Torture was common especially during 'struggle sessions' in which individuals were forced into admitting they were scholars. It's estimated that at least thirty million people died during this time, either from starvation or ill-treatment and a lot of these were academics. I learned that Rumei's father had spent many years in jail, simply because he was a teacher of English. His wife, also a retired teacher, was a delightful little lady, and although she spoke no English, always reserved a special welcome for me whenever I visited. They didn't have much, but what they had they shared with me and I loved them dearly.

Central Chinese Television produced only five minutes of news in English at nine in the morning. The rest was in Chinese, as one would expect. Some documentary programmes concerning animals and the countryside were easy to follow, but the half hour 'soaps', which my neighbours loved, were impossible for me to understand in my early days. Fortunately, my short-wave radio survived the journey within my rucksack, and I could pick up a multitude of programmes from many parts of the world. Unfortunately, it could only get snatches of BBC Worldwide and Voice of America. I guessed the nearby mountain ranges and tall buildings blocked the reception. There was nothing I could do to improve it.

My six CDs were played almost every day and soon became more than familiar. All in all, I had little entertainment of any kind. I made a calendar and notes to record the days and events, and sat back and waited for something or anything to happen. I had no telephone so couldn't contact my family or even my fellow volunteers who, by now, were scattered all over mainland China carrying out their teaching roles. My nerves were gradually being shredded and my patience was running thin. At times, I wondered if I could possibly survive and began to think I had made a terrible mistake. Sometimes I felt I would go mad if my circumstances didn't change. Activities were limited and I was desperate to escape. The Foreign Affairs Department at the Medical College appeared to have forgotten me, so I was overjoyed to hear a tentative knock on my door one morning. I opened it to see the smiling face of Chen Wen Jia, the twelve-year-old who lived in the flat above. He was slim and his black hair was in a close crew cut. He wore a blue T-shirt over jeans and the toes of his shoes were scuffed.

"Can I help?" He asked hesitantly as I invited him in. "I empty your trash can," he said, and henceforth took on the daily run to the rat-infested rubbish heap.

His mother, Yi Jiang, was a nurse and his father, Chen Li, an accountant. Eight-year old Chen Wen Hao was the youngest member of the family. He was full of mischief and I rarely saw him without a cheeky grin. It wasn't long before this family became essential to my well-being. They taught me many things, including the strict rules regarding the one-child policy. I was to learn that this particular family had two children because, although the father was Han Chinese, the mother was of the Bai ethnic minority group which allowed them to have more than one child. Many happy days were spent with this delightful family visiting Yi Jiang's home village, sailing on the beautiful lake nearby and learning about rural family life. Chen Wen Jia was learning American English at school and every day he brought his homework for me to check. Before long, his friends came as well and soon I began to get pleasure from my new self-made role as English coach to these lively children. These sessions had a dual function, English homework for them and Mandarin lessons for me. I think they also saved my sanity as they gave me a purpose, a feeling of being needed in my lonely existence.

Yang Kaishun, the doctor who was caring for my injuries was a short, slim man with an engaging smile. In his early thirties, and always immaculately dressed, he was the sole occupier of the block of flats adjacent to mine. He was studying for another degree and as his spoken English was limited, he brought his documents for me to hear him read on a regular basis. We joked as he wrestled with the grammar and pronunciation, but he was a good student and quickly improved. He explained that all his papers had to be written in English and, although he had studied the language at school, he had never been taught the spoken word. He was keen to improve this skill and, as he had no patients to care for, we spent many hours together perfecting his English. He was proud of his parents who, poor as they were, had struggled to send him to university. He was proud of his achievement.

One day he invited me to his flat for a meal. The kitchen was furnished with a small table and four low stools. On a worktop stood a single gas jet burner attached to a gas cylinder, a wok, a kettle, a few utensils and half a dozen bowls. The living room was empty and one bedroom was kitted out with a double bunk bed and a small desk, which stood nearby. This orthopaedic consultant sat and studied on the lower part of the bed during the day and slept on it at night. The top bunk was littered with his few possessions. During his spare time, he made furniture in preparation for when his wife, a nurse, and their little girl joined him. They had been forced to remain in his hometown some one hundred kilometres away and he was pulling every string to get them to Xiaguan, but it wasn't easy. I had begun to learn about the forced separations that so many Chinese families endured. When I thought of the 'luxuries' that were provided for me in my accommodation I felt lucky. I wasn't exactly pampered, but I had more than most people around me.

Although these new friends were my immediate salvation, on some days I felt miserable and began to yearn for western company, if only for general conversation and humour. I ticked off the days on my homemade calendar, listened to Phil Collins, Freddie Mercury and Eric Clapton again and again and kept a diary. At that moment, there wasn't much I could do to alter things and so I buried my head in my guide book to learn about local life and the ancient city of Dali, which lay some fourteen km away.

Chapter 8

With the hospital still under construction, the leaders decided I would be teaching sixty senior nurses in a classroom situation with some use of a practical room for demonstrations. They didn't consult me but obviously felt the British models of nursing practice would be beneficial. I was quite satisfied with this, after all I had come to try and improve the inpatient care and a start had to be made somewhere. The course participants were to be ferried in from local hospitals and clinics. The school year was divided into two terms of seventeen weeks duration because of the link with the medical college. At the end of each term I would send a report to the VSO office in Beijing

Rumei and I sat for hours planning the sessions. We had some interesting times, for although she had an excellent command of English, she was an English teacher and knew absolutely nothing about nursing. Having never worked with an interpreter I wondered if my message would get across. Only time would tell. In a short while I was going to meet the nurses, who were all mature and qualified, although I wouldn't be teaching them until I was more mobile.

Finally, the day came and as I entered the classroom, a great hush descended and sixty pairs of dark eyes focused on me. "Hello everyone," I said, hoping the tremble in my voice wasn't audible as I took a seat next to Rumei.

Miss Li made a formal introduction and the nurses, all female, replied with a well-practised, "Ello and welcome."

The professional guidance I'd hoped for and expected from this head nurse, Miss Li, didn't materialise. In fact, she seemed hell bent on preventing me from doing anything constructive. She sat with a face like thunder and shouted at my every suggestion. There were moments when I swear wisps of smoke crept from her nostrils. I began to feel that this woman didn't want any input from me and maybe this was why she had behaved so badly on our journey from Kunming. She was obviously in total charge of all nursing proceedings and was resentful. She stomped around the room, slammed books on the table and shouted in Chinese. Her behaviour reminded me of a dominant lioness who felt her cubs were being threatened. What was her problem? There was no way I could know, so I grabbed my books and left the room utterly confused. Someone, somewhere, had requested guidance from a British nurse and it most certainly wasn't this woman. I could only surmise she'd lost face where I was concerned and I knew I had met my own personal 'dragon'. There was no doubt in my mind that coming to terms with local practices and beliefs was going to be a difficult process and I knew I had a great deal to learn about the workings of the Chinese mind. Even 'please' or 'thank you' was rarely said; there was no need in a country where everyone was equal, I was told. What chance did I have? This was not going to be easy.

Prior to my UK departure, I had made many enquiries regarding China and its nursing practices. Little information was available at that time, but I did discover that the Chinese Nursing body was not a member of the World Council of Nurses. I had no idea on the type of training these nurses had received so some sort of a relationship with this head nurse was essential. There were so many questions that needed answering. Also some guidelines of what was expected of me during my teaching sessions would have been more than useful, but it was obvious this particular 'dragon' was not going to co-operate and once more I felt lonely and vulnerable.

Back in my flat I was in a quandary and wasn't sure what I should do, but when Rumei arrived some ten minutes later I'd recovered most of my reasoning. She put her arm around me and smiled. "Maybe you shouldn't have walked out like that, but I'm not surprised. You are very different from us in so many ways and I know everything is strange for you. I couldn't help you during the meeting, but I'm here now", and with that we put our heads together to consider my next move.

She explained the workings of the hospital hierarchy to me and her knowledge and support was invaluable. I expected everything to be different but as nurses were we really poles apart? Or was Ms Li simply trying to make life difficult for me?

"Has anyone ever asked these nurses what they would like to learn?" I asked Rumei.

"We can't ask them" was her shocked reply. "Students are never consulted. It's just not done here."

"Well," I said, "this will be a first, and if you will help me, I'll have a go."

If the 'dragon' wouldn't help I would have to find out what the nurses expected from me, so I prepared a questionnaire. Rumei translated it and made sixty-two hand-written copies in Chinese. There would be one for each of the nurses, one for the 'dragon' and one for the hospital chief.

With a mischievous grin, she turned to me. "I'm going now to try to arrange a get-together with the hospital leaders. See you soon."

She returned within half an hour. "We've got a meeting at six o'clock this evening. You'll have to be careful how you approach this matter. It's an unusual request that you are making, but you know I'll help as much as I can."

The gathering ran smoothly, even though the 'dragon' never took her eyes off me I felt satisfied and motivated. In due course, the surprised students replied to my questionnaire and their needs were quite clear: they would appreciate an update of their clinical nursing skills and an insight into Western living, both in the nursing field and life in general. I thanked my lucky stars that I had brought the Royal Marsden Manual of Clinical Nursing with me and for the next few weeks that book became my bible. I had won the day, but the battle continued and the 'dragon' was not amused.

Chapter 9

Two weeks into my placement, I couldn't sleep. For the first time since arriving in China I felt deeply depressed and spent half the time snivelling and worrying about everything and anything. One morning, after my little friend Chen Wen Jia had brought me my breakfast, I sat with my head in my hands. I knew that too much time alone with no western company was my problem. The difference of opinion with the head nurse hadn't helped, and without Rumei visiting when she could I think I might have cracked. The plaster on my leg wasn't quite dry and I hadn't a clue what was going on around me. This immobility was a new experience and I didn't like it. My kitchen and living room had become a prison.

What on earth had possessed me to leave my work, home, friends and family? Did I really think I would cope, or was I mad? I remembered my three children and their families; I had four beautiful grandsons in England. We had never lived in each other's pockets, but we shared so many things in life, both good and bad. Now I needed their company. I wanted somebody I knew really well to sit and have a good old fashioned talk with me, someone to whom I could pour out my heart. To compound the problem I couldn't even pick up the phone to contact a friend. I had no computer and therefore no email. The Foreign Affairs Department had taken my passport to obtain a work permit and a resident's card. The mail seemed to take forever, meaning I had nothing to do but sit and wait. Money was also very tight adding to the feeling of isolation.

I had always considered myself to be the 'eternal optimist' but now I was having grave doubts. Even though I had my homemade calendar, I began to lose days. Somehow, I had to change things and pull myself together. How I wished I could start my teaching programme, although where I would actually start I didn't yet know.

On her usual visit, poor Rumei got the full blast of my frustrations. She was alarmed but it worked wonders and before the end of that day a telephone had been installed enabling me to make in-country calls to some of my new VSO teacher friends. Arrangements were also made for me to eat in a small roadside café just outside the hospital confines. I felt I was being released from my prison at last and I looked forward to a meal with Rumei that evening. It was quite a long walk to the café and although the crutches were a help, the road was in a primitive state. I carefully picked my way between the rocks, potholes and litter. Once there, I was consumed with a bout of gastronomic cowardice and settled for an omelette. An eventful day had passed and slowly, slowly, I began to climb back into an optimistic frame of mind.

I usually woke to the clink of glass as a farmer delivered milk to the flat where a small child lived. Today, more than anything, I wanted a drink of the white stuff and left my flat to

47

buy some. When I saw the milk was in something suspiciously like a used intravenous drip bottle, probably discarded from a local hospital or clinic, I changed my mind. I swear the rubber stopper had been used as I could see the tiny hole that the needle always made when an intravenous drip was given. Somehow, I didn't fancy drinking the milk when I considered what kind of mixture had preceded it! I could have boiled it, but because I was living at an altitude of nearly two thousand metres, I wasn't certain the milk would be sterilised. I knew there was less air pressure at elevation, which reduces the boiling point, and I wanted to be safe, not sorry.

Building was continuing on the new hospital. I could see it was a long way from completion and probably wouldn't be ready for another six months at the earliest. Thankfully, my mobility was improving daily, my plaster was almost dry and I began to feel excited at the thought of exploring the city in the near future.

At midday, I was surprised by a welcome visit from Bryan, an Englishman who lived with his Italian wife and two children in Shaping, a village on the lakeside some thirty kilometres away. He had heard of my solitary plight from medical college friends. As we sat and chatted I was astonished to learn of two Australians who lived and worked in the teachers' training college just a paddy field away from me. My spirits soared. Why the Foreign Affairs Department hadn't given me such vital information I would never know.

Later, Yang Kaishun, the doctor who had renewed the plaster on my foot, arrived with his books under his arm. We spent an interesting hour or so just talking about the hospital. He told me more about his family. He obviously missed them a great deal. "I study most days. It keeps my thinking positive. I shall be glad when the hospital opens its doors to patients as I need to keep up to date with my surgery." he explained. He went on to tell me about some textbooks, Campbell's Operative Techniques, which he desperately needed. I promised to do a search on the cost and availability of them.

When he got up to leave, I went to the window to wave him off. In the distance, I could see two little girls playing with some chalk. They drew what resembled a hopscotch frame. They were laughing and whispering. It took me back to my own early days. I wondered about Yang Kaishun's childhood, but he never spoke about it. It wasn't until I came to China that I appreciated the idyllic childhood I'd experienced, compared with the majority of people I had met in Xiaguan so far.

Chapter 10

My cast was dry at last and Yang Kaishun fitted a hand-made wooden rocker to the base of my plaster from a design I had drawn. A strip of rubber from an old tyre was used as a sole and it meant I could discard my crutches and be almost normal again. It was heaven to be mobile and my mood lifted immediately. Poor Yang Kaishun wasn't quite so cheerful because I had received information on the textbooks he wanted. The price meant they were totally out of his reach.

"It doesn't matter," he sighed. "It was just a dream. Maybe one day I'll be able to buy them. See you soon." And he was gone.

With my new mobility, I was able to work. I needed to get involved with something, anything, to save my sanity. In my nursing career, I'd had plenty of teaching experience and I was keen to start my sessions. They would take place three afternoons a week for the rest of the term, some fourteen weeks. It didn't sound much, but each lesson had to last for three hours. The preparation would last even longer with the vast amount of planning and writing involved, and I was still without a computer. A long time ago I discovered that teaching is always more successful if you select the subjects the students prefer, so at a meeting I asked the sixty nurses which of the many nursing procedures they would like to update. They were delighted and presented me with a list of topics. Rumei and I worked side-by-side. Her expertise and company were more than welcome. I was working again but it wasn't long before I realised I wouldn't have much freedom on the content of the topics, as every presentation was vetted by not only the 'dragon', but also the hospital chiefs.

And so, the day came when Rumei and I entered the classroom to present a teaching session. I was excited but at the same time a few butterflies had crept into my stomach. I had given presentations to many different audiences in the past, but this was going to be very different. Fortunately, my dragon was not around and the nurses were smiling as once more they all stood up and said "Ello" in unison. This meeting was one of great discovery for me as we had dedicated the first two hours to finding out as much as possible about these women, such as names and places of work, and a little of their family situations. We were all senior nurses, so our working backgrounds were unsurprisingly similar and I took many notes. With the thirty-odd double seated desks bolted firmly to the floor in neat rows there wouldn't be any opportunity for small informal chatty circles which I had always found extremely beneficial in the past. No, my translator and I would be standing in the front of the blackboard with pieces of dusty chalk in our hands, just as my primary school teacher, Mrs Evans, had done all those years ago in East Allington, a small village in South Devon.

Every session brought something new and I was more than surprised to discover my class had a monitor. This person, a student, was a 'party member' and would report the content of my lecture to the hierarchy. I never knew who it was, but it was a clear reminder for me never to stray into politics, religion or even world events. I was in China and not entirely free to speak my private thoughts. Sometimes, to fill in a thirty-minute gap, we would talk about our personal experiences relating to nursing. It was difficult and I quickly realised these nurses were unable, or unwilling, to express their thoughts and feelings, particularly those involving infant mortality and abortion. I wondered if the Marxist philosophy had somehow suppressed their personalities and thoughts, and I felt sad for them.

Work-wise, with the head nurse keeping well out of my way, I felt I had won some independence. The weeks flew by and I was encouraged by the regular feedback Rumei provided. My glossy British nursing publications, which came by mail, were very popular, especially the articles which contained explicit coloured photographs. On one occasion, I selected an article written by three English nurses who had lost their babies in infancy. These women had been able to express the grief experienced, not only by themselves as new mothers, but also the feelings of their partners or husbands and families. They spoke of the professional help that had been made available to them during these sad times and how they coped when finally, able to resume their nursing careers. This session really brought these Chinese nurses to life. They came out of the shadows and couldn't stop talking. Many had tears in their eyes. The talented Rumei switched effortlessly between the two languages, which not only enabled the sessions to flow, but also provided a good insight into the diverse and often difficult lives of these women who were nurses; just like me.

They were taken aback to discover many British nurses moved from job to job for various reasons, including promotion, and even more surprised to find that men also became nurses. In that part of China nursing was entirely a female occupation. They told me how, when she had completed her training, a Chinese nurse was sent to a unit, usually in her hometown. She would remain there, doing the same job until she retired. I was learning so much from these women, but at this stage I had no idea how they carried out their work. I was going to have to bide my time. One day I hoped to be able to go onto the wards, even though I knew it would only be in an observational capacity, and it was something to look forward to. I quickly settled in to the routine and began to look forward to being with the nurses as they worked. Rumei was excited by my approach and in a few weeks this girl was not only my advisor and carer, but also my best friend.

Six weeks after my phone was connected I got a call from one of my sons to tell me my dear friend's husband had died. Margaret and I were extremely close, having been friends since we were eighteen. I felt I should have been with her and phoned a couple of times to offer my love and support. My phone charges were taken out of my salary at the end of the month and when I received less than half my meagre earnings from Miss Li, the head nurse, she sneered and said 'ello, ello, ello,' and cackled like an old crow. I badly wanted to mimic her in derision, but that would achieve nothing so I just walked away. What a compassionate lady I thought and wondered where the nurse in her had gone!

Then, after six weeks of constant planning and teaching I became depressed again and wanted to stay in bed. I felt thoroughly wretched and miserable. Even though I had half expected this despair to hit me for a second time I was slow in recognising it, and even slower in coming to grips with the situation. Somehow, I had to keep going and motivate myself to climb out of the big black hole I was in.

Contributing to my distress was the fact that I couldn't pick up my phone and chat to an English friend, due to the cost. Once more I began to have doubts in myself. I must have been foolish to think I would ever survive in a place like this. I was lonely and craved western company. There was no real friendship with the Chinese nurses I knew; they were great girls, but culturally so very different from me and we did have a serious communication problem when Rumei wasn't around. Because they were unable to express their emotions they seemed startled when I told them how I was feeling. I wondered what sort of training they had received and whether they looked after each other and sometimes cried together when times were tough. This happened in every British hospital I'd been employed in, and now I was trying to live a life quite alien to me. I was finding it hard, but had no choice. I would have to get on with things or get out, and I didn't want to do that, not when I'd come this far. Somehow life had to go on, and desolate as I felt, I had to get a grip on the situation. In the end, it was probably my sheer stubbornness and tenacity that enabled me to get by.

Chapter 11

Life wasn't all studying and teaching and when my second plaster cast was removed I felt well and ready to go exploring in my free time. Most evenings were spent with a number of children who lived within the hospital complex, playing five-a-side football on a large area of concrete. I loved this. These boys and girls were great fun and the exercise certainly kept me fit. The kids would pretend to be David Beckham, whom they called Beck-Ham. He was idolised by all the boys and girls. During our rest periods, these youngsters would give me language lessons and simple local expressions. They taught me swear words and would fall around laughing when I copied them. I became an expert in telling the time and counting. They made sure I pronounced the words properly by making me repeat the difficult syllables over and over, never letting me off the hook. During the quieter moments, they spoke of their personal experiences, both happy and sad and I began to feel accepted by this little community that had become so special to me.

Fortunately, walking was no problem, and with a morning free I decided to visit the local market. It didn't take me long to realise that I was not equipped for this experience. I ventured into the fruit and meat market and pushed my way down the narrow gap in the middle. A teeming mass of noisy humanity laughed and pointed at me. It was almost as if I was an alien with some sort of celebrity status simply because I was so different. Children pointed and giggled and said 'Ello,' while their parents taught their snotty nosed kids to say, *'Lao Wei'* which meant outsider or foreigner. I soon discovered a lot could be implied from the delivery and intonation of those two words.

A young man with roughly cut, spiky hair and red betel-nut stained broken teeth confronted me. He was selling large grey maggots which were alive and wriggling in a bowl. He thrust a handful a few inches from my face. "Yuk." I said and we stared into each other's eyes until eventually I backed away. The maggots were no doubt full of nutrition and were probably tasty, but I was not that hungry.

Many of the older traders were dressed in olive green suits or dark blue Mao outfits, with fastenings up to the neck. Back in the fifties and sixties, when the 'Great Helmsman,' or Chairman Mao, was in power, both men and women wore these clothes as a symbol of equality and many of the older people still wore this type of garment. These sellers looked exhausted. I was to learn later they'd probably left their homes in the early hours to make the journey down the mountains. I saw loads of beautiful fresh vegetables, some of which I didn't recognise and bought some cabbage, carrots, onions and coriander before fighting my way to the meat counters. Dog meat had been jointed and placed in large wicker baskets. Fluffy tails had been left dangling off the rumps so the breed could be recognised. I knew these animals had been bred for many years for their meat, and not only in China, but it didn't help to see it in front of me for the first time. I didn't spend a lot of time looking at it. Life for some of these animals was surely dreadfully different here. I was upset and thought about dogs I had owned, remembering the good times we had spent together. They were so much a part of my family and when they died it was almost akin to losing a close friend. It was quite a relief to know that some Chinese acquaintances who had little pet dogs, loved them and spoilt them rotten, so it wasn't all bad.

Eventually I found a pork counter and selected a fillet that was warm and soft to my touch. I felt I had to handle it as everyone else was doing the same! There were no fridges in the market and freshly killed meat had been placed on long wooden slabs. Sometimes it looked as if it was still alive and moving because it was covered in flies, and to make matters worse, two dead rats were lying sprawled out on the ground less than three metres away. It certainly wasn't inviting and my mind raced into overtime when I considered what sort of disease I might catch, but whatever, I had to eat and knew I could never become a vegetarian. Refrigeration in most homes was still a bit of a novelty at this time and most people shopped twice daily for their food.

Around the corner I found stalls with dozens of padded bras, lacy nylon knickers, brightly coloured cheap tops, miniskirts and shoes. All the goods were in small sizes for tiny people, making me with my clothes size twelve feel like a giant.

All around me people hawked, coughed and spat as if the whole world depended on it and the road looked like a communal spittoon. It wasn't so much the hawk and eventual cough, which could be heard some fifty metres away, that worried me so much, but where was the sputum going to land? And there was nowhere to take cover. Others held a finger to a nostril and blew the contents onto the ground before repeating the episode on the other side. Any residual nasal mucus was neatly removed with dirty fingers and wiped on the nearest available object. Both these bodily functions were dealt with in a manner achieved after what must have been years of concentration and practice. Suddenly, without ceremony, I was shoved out of the way to allow a white-coated man to pass. He was pushing a low trolley stacked with small cans. All around the sides were stuffed dead rats. I assumed he was selling rat poison, but experience had taught me never to take anything for granted. Who really knew what he was doing? The rats were a real menace locally and dead ones were common sights in gutters and corners. I learned there was a grave shortage of cats and people didn't seem to have them as pets. Sadly, cats did make a tasty meal for many local folk and, for a horrifying moment I wondered if I'd already eaten cat-meat. I wouldn't know because most of the meat I ate in any cafe was almost ground to a pulp. The cat skins were useful too as they made lovely soft fluffy covers for the pot animals that were made locally. For a few moments I felt sad, as on reflection, having cats around had improved my quality of life. I tried to put unpleasant thoughts out of my mind as I headed towards the fruit sellers who, I was to discover, always put two extra oranges into my bag, whether I wanted them or not!

My first lone outing was like a physical and mental assault course for which I'd had no training. I'd witnessed poverty on a level I'd never met before but simultaneously experienced kindness and consideration from these same individuals. I felt completely drained as I trailed slowly back to my flat.

On making enquiries into the constant hawking, spitting and coughing that seemed to occur all the time, I learned that the westerners' habit of using tissues to blow their noses in was considered by the local population to be the most terribly dirty habit imaginable, made even worse when the snotty tissue was returned to a pocket. To me it was good news and if I kept a few tissues in all my pockets I would hopefully never have my pockets picked. I was learning all the time!

My market visit had been quite an experience, but didn't distract me from wanting to see more of the city, so a few days later I explored the hospital vicinity with my twelve-year-old friend Chen Wen Jia, who lived in the flat above me. He chattered non-stop and was great company. Xiaguan, also known as New Dali, appeared to be a dreary, characterless city which had been recently constructed. The dismal grey buildings were put up in rectangular shaped blocks surrounded by roads which all seemed to be at right angles. I looked for landmarks on this my first trip. It proved to be difficult. On every street corner, there seemed to be an electrical shop selling items identical to the last. If I selected an eating-house with chairs and tables on the pavement, a comparable one could be found on the next corner. Slowly, I familiarised myself with my new habitat aided by my little friend, and began to feel at home.

Rumei's father told me that the more fortunate city dwellers lived in what to me were depressing, colourless blocks of flats attached to work units. They had employment and a purpose, no matter how small. Most of the open stairwells I saw were cluttered with items ranging from bikes, boxes and plants to the odd noisy cockerel housed in strong cardboard box. These unfortunate birds were fed with household scraps and idled their days away waiting for a family celebration to herald their demise.

Later, as I grew more adventurous and went further afield, I saw primitive conditions in poorer parts of the city. Whole families housed themselves in a tiny shed or a corrugated iron lean-to. They existed, crammed together in proximities which would be unimaginable in the West. Understandably they had achieved a high level of tolerance. Their tiny cramped conditions led me to believe it was little wonder that they seemed to be continually on the move, with families walking along the streets in what appeared to be a slow Chinese saunter. A few would enter the shops to look around, but mostly they appeared to be meandering, oblivious to everything and everyone.

Work for these people was difficult to find. A lucky few had small horses and carts or three-wheeled cycles with a trailer attached, but for most it was a crude handcart. Owners of these, both men and women gritted their teeth and heaved huge loads of furniture and white goods or enormous pyramids of polystyrene through the streets. They had to navigate around massive lumps of concrete and dog-sized potholes and, at the same time, inhale fumes that belched from passing trucks and buses. They had a hard existence and it showed in their faces. Every road I took was festooned by a tangled mass of overhead electrical and telephone cables. They seemed to be attached to the corners of any building that happened to be there. Who could know which cable belonged to which building? And some hung only a few feet above my head. I wondered what our British health and safety bosses would think of the hotchpotch clumps of multi-coloured wires!

Chapter 12

On a day off, I decided to walk the two kilometres or so to the city to post some mail and collect a package from the Post Office. I had received a slip of paper from the Foreign Affairs Department telling me a parcel awaited collection.

I walked through the gates and headed down the road from the hospital. It was a fairly new area and was beginning to take shape as building progressed; it was dusty and untidy, but becoming more alive and noisy. Numerous little food shops and cafes had opened and people were moving into nearby flats. A farmer was encouraging his herd of seven skinny cows to hurry up the steep hill, but these docile animals seemed to be far more interested in rummaging about in the large bins for cabbage leaves or any other tasty morsel they could find. I passed a fire station on my left and saw what appeared to be military personnel cleaning and polishing fire engines and tenders until they must have been able to see their reflections in the bodywork.

At the road junction, I turned right and continued along a rough pavement by the side of a made-up road. So many and varied actions were taking place in such a small area. A beautiful girl was sitting on the pavement, washing her shiny, long black hair in a huge enamel bowl. I saw two youths in greasy overalls fixing an engine and in the next unit four men were drilling and hammering metal window frames. On a street corner, a man with a towel around his neck was sitting on a low stool shaving and washing in a chipped enamel bowl. He held a small round mirror in his hand. In numerous small hole-in-the-wall eating places, groups of men were laughing and talking as they sat on low stools and slurped their noodles and washed them down with Dali beer.

I heard the Bridal Chorus chimes as a dustcart approached, its bells telling everyone to bring out their rubbish. In a flash, five or six scruffy, dirty street-kids appeared and took turns to dive into the back of the truck to retrieve plastic bottles and paper. They escaped just as the crusher was about to squash them. They packed their goodies in large plastic bags and carried them away, presumably to the recycling shed where they would sell whatever they could. From their appearance, they looked as if they made barely enough to survive. What could I do? Nothing really, except try not to be noticed as I pushed a few Yuan into a grubby little hand, empty of rubbish loot. On the way home, I wondered about these kids. Where did they live and who, if anyone, looked after them? I was curious and hoped to find out at some stage.

I reached the bridge and another absorbing scene unfolded. A cobbler was cutting up an old lorry tyre and expertly repairing boots with the treads; a young man was leaning over the parapet with an enamel mug of water in one hand and a toothbrush in the other, cleaning his teeth; a woman was toasting corn-on-the-cob over smoking charcoal for two children, who were clapping their hands in eagerness. Two women wearing dusty masks and dirty white overalls were slowly sweeping the wide street with large besom brooms. They deposited the rubbish in handcarts, which stood overflowing at the side of the road. The little open-air barber shops were crowded with middle aged men having their hair dyed. They sat under hairdryers with their ears covered with stained white plastic ear protectors, seemingly staring into space. Alongside them in a small cubby hole between the buildings young men were selling homemade feather dusters with long brown chicken-wing feathers attached to bamboo poles with sticky tape. I passed clothes shops blaring western music. At the entrances, rows of girls were clapping to the beat as they tried to encourage people to step inside and buy the highly coloured sequin speckled articles that lined the walls and rails inside.

More young men in groups of sixes and sevens had their arms wrapped around each other and were laughing and talking. On the other side of the road, girls were doing the same only giggling as well. There were no boy and girl couples to be seen. It seemed this was just not done. Scooters, with pillion passengers balanced precariously side-saddle, rushed by. I envied their sense of balance. I wouldn't have lasted for five minutes. Occasionally a small child clinging monkey-like to his scooter riding dad would pass me on the way to the local kindergarten. Every other person seemed to be yelling down a mobile phone, sharing their conversations with all and sundry. In that thirty-minute walk I had observed a corner of another world.

I finally reached the post office and squeezed towards the foreigners' counter prepared for the inevitable wait. The place was rowdy and crowded with people of all ages. Some were producing an assortment of articles for inspection by the postal staff and, after scrutiny, were cramming them into white canvas bags. The nimble-fingered ones were threading large needles with yarn and stitching the bags, ready for posting. Queuing was obviously unheard of and it was clearly a case of every man for himself. I joined them and eventually made it to the counter. When I produced my slip of paper for the package, I discovered that I had to pay a fee for storage and handling! But it was worth it. A gift from home was like manna from heaven and I held it close to my heart. My letters were duly weighed and I paid for the stamps. I elbowed my way to a table to seal the envelopes and attach the stamps with a dubious looking runny, gooey substance which passed for glue. I felt sticky and dirty and wanted to wash my hands but instead fought my way back to the man on the foreigners' counter and watched as he franked the stamps and put my precious letters in a bag for collection.

I had learned so much on this single trip my mind was in a whirl. I knew it wouldn't be long before I accepted it as the norm, very different from the activities on the Worcester streets

I knew so well. For me this was another life and at last I was beginning to feel part of it.

Every evening a strange phenomenon occurred in the city. As the light faded, an evening wind would thunder through a pass and hurtle down the mountainside with a sound like ball bearings rattling in a can. For a full three minutes, it moved everything not nailed down: papers, cigarette packets, cans, even glasses and plates. Doors and windows clattered and in its wake people were able to breathe what surely must have been sweet mountain air, savouring its purity. When the winds didn't blow, rain was usually on the way. It became a good weather forecast and I was reminded almost daily why this place was known locally as the 'windy city'.

A few days later, with the street kids weighing heavily on my mind, I asked the Foreign Affairs department if I could visit an orphanage or children's home at some time. "Yes, of course you can. We will arrange it and let you know." I was informed. But in the three years spent in Xiaguan this promise was never honoured and the only thing I could do was secretly hand over a few Yuan whenever I saw an unfortunate child. And there were so many.

Chapter 13

Six weeks after my arrival in Xiaguan I set off to visit the ancient city of Dali. My mission was two-fold. Firstly, I wanted to find Vicky and Ian, the Australians who had a placement in the nearby teachers' college, and secondly, I wanted to explore the city, with its ancient gates and temples. There was a spring in my step as I walked to the No 4 bus terminus in Xiaguan. I was excited and had no idea what to expect.

It was market day in Dali and the airless bus was packed with commuters. I squeezed into an empty seat near the front. My language skills were still poor, but as the bus only went as far as Dali, with a Chinese character I had memorised, I figured that nothing could go wrong. The uniformed conductress pushed her way between the passengers. She was unsmiling as she collected the fares before taking her place behind the driver where she could be in full control and make decisions as to who could, or could not ride on the bus. The wooden seats were hard and the road was full of potholes, but that didn't stop the little lady next to me putting her head on my shoulder and instantly falling asleep. This was a common occurrence on the local buses, but I never discovered how these same people were able to suddenly wake up and alight at the correct stop. This mystery has remained with me.

We rattled through the villages alongside Erhai Lake, passing fields of yellow rape and purple-flowering tobacco plants. At every stop people pushed their way onto the already filled bus, some with open buckets containing live fish, and others with tied hessian sacks containing squeaking puppies or piglets. We passed men working with stone-grinding machines. Some were piling the rocks into these contraptions with spades; others were shovelling the resulting sand into heaps and were grey with the resulting thick dust that swirled around them. Further along, stonemasons were carving elaborate patterns into marble headstones, which would be carried up the mountainside to graves when needed. Others worked on the granite or marble lions that I had seen adorning the occasional front door. Not one of these workers wore any eye or ear protection. Many of the houses lining the road were bedecked with bright yellow corncobs drying in the sun. Others had homemade hatbands, ribbons and metres of plaited straw that fluttered in the breeze; making straw hats was a fairly lucrative home industry for some.

Down a narrow street, women were laughing together as they carved intricate designs into wooden chairs, beds and screens in small hole-in-the-wall workshops. Groups of men in blue Mao suits sat on the steps outside these places, undoubtedly putting the world to rights. In the distance, I could see the ancient three-story building known as the South Gate of the city. Its impressive two-tiered red-tiled roof had eaves that curved heavenwards. It was adorned with colourful flags and was surrounded by traders selling marble memorabilia, batiks, tie-dye fabrics and cheap silver jewellery.

After the bus entered a short tunnel, passing beneath the South Gate, it ground to a halt in one of the beautiful old streets. I stepped on to the road and immediately fell in love with the sights and sounds around me.

A ghetto blaster on full decibels delivered the high-pitched, shrill voice of a female Chinese pop star as I passed a tiny kiosk. The lady owner tapped her foot and hummed along to the tune as she sold preserved fruits and multi-coloured homemade sweets. They looked so good I bought some to chew as I walked along. The traders in the crooked little wooden shops further down the street were puffing on their cigarettes and laughing together as they stacked their goods. They displayed so many items in heaps so high, that invariably the goods tumbled out on to the pavements.

The gold-coloured statue of a soldier, which stood some three metres high, was to the right of the entrance of the army barracks. I stopped short of taking a photo as I'd been warned I might have my film confiscated if I snapped anything remotely military, such was the paranoia of the officials.

Dali is an ancient city with a remarkable history that stretches back over 10,000 years. Many of the twenty-six ethnic groups of Yunnan Province live there, but it is the home of the Bai ethnic minority who roused most interest in me. Those I knew practised Buddhism. Communism didn't normally allow much room for religion, but these people, especially the women, were exceptionally strong. They ignored the rules brought in by Chairman Mao when he came to power in 1949 and defiantly continued the family traditions with great pride as had been done by their ancestors for centuries. Their elegant houses were mainly of wooden construction, with stone walled courtyards decorated with brightly coloured carvings and scenic paintings. The women looked striking as they went about their daily business wearing bright red side-fastening embroidered vests and multi-coloured aprons over white blouses and black trousers. Their headdresses were stunning as well, being mainly red and white with a band of embroidered pink camellias around the front edge. Their hair was coiled around the brim if they were married. Single girls had a long braid hanging over a shoulder.

It has long been accepted that this beautiful city is one of the last stops on the hippy trail in Southeast Asia. During my stay, it was common knowledge that all kinds of hallucinogenic drugs were freely available. Some were hidden in the back streets, yet others grew by the roadside. Often the same women who sold the tie-dye fabrics and silver jewellery sold the drugs and they knew who to approach, usually westerners. Foreign travellers would arrive after hiking through India, Nepal and the Golden Triangle. Most were positively skinny with ragged Indian style clothing hanging from emaciated bodies. Although this city was a mere fourteen kilometres from Xiaguan, it was so different, both in its approach to foreigners and to life in general. People here seemed more relaxed and hospitable. I could feel the calm, tranquil ambience as I ambled along, and I treasured it.

Finally, I found Huguo Lu, or Foreigners' Street, so called because of the multitude of cafes, guesthouses and touristy shops. Along this street I saw western tourists sitting in small groups around pavement cafes. They were enjoying the local Dali beer and gazing at the magical snow-capped peaks of the Cangshan Mountains, while trying to ignore the tie-dye and silver sellers who were pestering them. Around the corner I discovered Jack's café, a place where people met and ate in a congenial atmosphere. This hostelry was to become my all-time favourite eating place during my three-year stay. Jack was polishing his motorbike near the entrance to his bar. He was Chinese, in his mid-twenties, had a good physique and was eye-catching in his black leathers. A red bandana was tied around his head and his long black hair was tied into a ponytail.

"Hi," he said, as he followed me into the bar. "This is my girlfriend, Stella. She's from Dali, like me, and runs a small pizza bar round the corner. You two get to know each other while I wash my hands. Then I'll be with you."

Stella was a slim, pretty twenty-three-year-old with an engaging smile. The short hairstyle suited her small round face and her eyes shone as she told me excitedly about the bar which she'd just opened. In that instant I felt they were a lovely couple, they seemed so happy in each other's company. Jack joined us. "You're English, aren't you?" he said. "I bet you'd love a coffee. Yeah?" With that, he made three drinks and we sat down and chatted.

I told them I was working at the new hospital in Xiaguan and wanted to find the Australian couple. "I know them," he said, "I think they'll be in the Coca Cola Café with Xiang Xia, the girl who runs it. Go down Foreigners' Street, over the crossroads and you'll find it on your left. I know there's not much in Xiaguan for the foreigners who live there, but remember you're always welcome in my cafe. My brother, Tim, is starting an internet service soon and I have a library of sorts in the corner over there. Hikers leave or swap their books and I've got a good supply of English classics, novels and travelling tales. You can borrow any of them. I also try to cook western food. See if there's anything you'd like on the menu and I'll prepare it for you."

Jack's command of English was near perfect and he came across as if he didn't have a worry in the world. He told me a visiting English teacher had given them English names several years ago and they were quite happy about it. I felt comfortable with him and Stella and joined them for a meal of egg and chips with homemade bread followed by their special chocolate cake and ice cream. I left them, promising a return visit in a few days.

At the bottom of Foreigners' Street, I spotted what was the Coca-Cola café, recently renamed The Yunnan Café, and inside I saw two smiling western faces.

"Hi. I'm Peggy from the new hospital and you must be Vicky and Ian. I've wanted to meet you for some time and I'm really pleased now that I have."

Vicky, who was tall and slight, looked good in her black trousers and cotton blouse. Her long blonde hair was tied back off her attractive face. Ian was slim as well, and wore a red T-shirt over blue jeans. They were vegetarians and 'earth lovers' and looked every bit a young picture-book couple.

"G'day gal, it's good to meet you," said Ian. "Come and join us. We've taught English in different parts of China for eight years. We've been here for a year now, and Dali is a beautiful place."

Their knowledge of the people, culture and language was so interesting I could have listened for hours. After much tea drinking and talking they invited me to visit them at the teachers training college that evening. It was a short distance from the hospital where I lived.

I was really happy to find people with similar thought processes to my own. I could relate to them in a western way and finally, I felt a new life was beginning.

As dusk approached I left the hospital grounds by one of the rear gates and found it guarded by a wizened little man who appeared to live in a small shed nearby. He looked as if he could do with a good square meal but seemed happy enough and nodded as I walked through the open gate.

It took twenty minutes to walk through the paddy fields to the teachers' college. I threaded my way along muddy, watery paths until I reached neat rows of narrow grassy banks that separated the paddies. Large green frogs jumped over the muddy barriers in front of me and their noisy bands ensured I wouldn't be lonely on my journey. On arrival, I reported to the guards. I was expected, and they phoned my new friends, who came to meet me.

The whole college looked unkempt and dilapidated. It had odd extensions protruding from many of the flats. These space enhancers were made from glass, wood and corrugated iron and looked strange. I quickly realised how fortunate I was to have a new flat with a western bathroom. Vicky and Ian's accommodation consisted of two bedrooms, a living room and a kitchen. A squat toilet was situated in a tiny room off the balcony behind the kitchen area. The bath actually stood in the kitchen and was surrounded by the gas ring, cooking utensils and kitchen sink. We chatted for hours over a tasty vegetarian meal washed down with Dali beer and I looked at their impressive, colourful collection of photos taken locally. I wondered if I would be able to achieve the same high quality. Time would tell.

We made arrangements for an early visit to Kunming, the capital city. I was delighted as my wish to explore this fascinating city had been whetted when I first arrived and now I was to have such pleasant company.

At the end of the evening they walked with me to the hospital where we found the guard's room in darkness. It took a few minutes of shouting and knocking before my shrivelled little friend appeared in his vest and long-johns to let me through the locked gates. With the aid of my torch I finally returned to my flat where eventually I climbed into my bed feeling happier than I had done for months

The following weeks were busy. I planned and wrote lectures and gave them to Rumei for translation. Our teaching sessions were being well received and I was growing in confidence. The thought of returning to Kunming with my new friends for a short weekend break gave me a real lift, and my depression had disappeared.

Chapter 14

A week after our first encounter, I met Ian and Vicky in Dali to book our seats on the Thursday overnight bus to Kunming. We didn't have work on Fridays, so we would be able to enjoy a long weekend away.

Every evening dozens of buses travelled from the depot in Xiaguan to Kunming, a journey of some four hundred kilometres, departing at about eight pm. Where the busses were concerned it was always a bit of a lottery with the sleeper beds, as many of the vehicles were old and dirty. Experience had taught my new friends that it was always better to start the journey from Dali and travel via Xiaguan with local drivers whose vehicles were reasonably clean and tidy. Vicky told me there would be food and a comfort stop about eleven o'clock in Chu Xiong, a small town en-route; otherwise it would be a non-stop ride. She also advised me to take some water as this particular expedition always varied in time because of the roadworks, but she thought we might make it in about fifteen hours. I was really excited and could hardly wait for Thursday evening to come.

Some time ago, a well-travelled friend had recommended that when in a foreign land, the tyres on any vehicle should be inspected for tread. A quick check on the driver should be made as well to check if he or she was sober before going on any journey. Alas, there was little hope of carrying out such an inspection in China, so on the Thursday evening when the overnight bus arrived to take us to Kunming I boarded with some trepidation. These vehicles had a facility for sleeping forty people, with double bunk-beds erected on either side of the narrow gangway.

At eight pm precisely we boarded with the a few other passengers and headed for our first stop at Xiaguan. We had booked our beds immediately behind the driver and his mate, so I felt reasonably safe. I was a little concerned though about my bed-mate, as the space was so small and the duvets and pillows were more than a bit grubby. Nevertheless, I straightened the covers, put my bag at my feet and chatted to my friends about Kunming. I only earned a small salary, so it was a real treat to spread my wings and do a little exploring of this lovely city I'd seen briefly on my arrival, and I congratulated myself on my good fortune to be with these two experienced people.

As we all settled in the driver switched on a noisy video at full decibels and everyone began shouting at each other as they chewed their sunflower seeds and spat out the husks. Most were making the journey in their work clothes, which had reached the point when they needed washing, and removed their shoes. After the Chinese passengers had closed most of the windows, lit cigarettes and had a good hawk, cough and a spit on the floor, we were away. At Xiaguan Bus Station a small crowd was waiting. It wasn't long before I discovered a young girl had been allocated the other half of my bed. There was some animated chatter about the *'Lao Wei'* or foreigner, but eventually she grunted acceptance and took her place beside me next to the window. I watched in amazement as small children were squeezed into tiny spaces between their parents as they settled in their bunks. The narrow gangway became crammed with an assortment of heavy cases, bags, taped cardboard boxes along with an assortment of motor components, including heavy metal leaf-springs. I said a little prayer and hoped we wouldn't have an emergency on the way.

The road hadn't changed much since I arrived a few weeks ago and our driver swerved and slammed on the brakes as he looked for ways around the obstacles ahead of him. Being dark we couldn't see the scenery, but perhaps it was as well because I had seen it all before when I first arrived and didn't really want to be reminded of the sheer drops down the mountainside. The two drivers chatted happily to each other, seemingly oblivious to the hullabaloo around them. When the babies needed to relieve themselves, their fathers held them out in the gangway, between the cardboard boxes and leaf springs, where they performed admirably. If anything, solid was produced it was wrapped in paper and thrown through the nearest window. There were no nappies or potties in this part of the world. The babies' pants had convenient slits in them which must have been damned chilly during the winter months! My bed-mate spent much of the time with her head hanging out the window, trying unsuccessfully to control her travel sickness.

At midnight, the bus drew to a halt in Chu Xiong. The men clambered over the cluttered gangway, jumped off, shot to the back of the bus and had a communal pee. When the coast was clear, I followed the women and to my great relief we all did the same. When in Rome, you do as the Romans do, no matter how you feel; privacy didn't seem to exist here. Anyway, after two months I had completely lost my inhibitions regarding the use of toilet facilities. I was quite happy to follow the masses and soon we were clambering back on board.

The lights were turned off, the video player was silent and we all settled down for a couple of hours sleep. We reached Kunming fourteen hours later and alighted with that horrible unwashed feeling that was to become all too familiar when travelling around China. At the bus station, I squeezed past a lady cleaner and made for the toilet. I was pleased to find this particular one not only had a door, but a bolt as well. Aha, a little privacy at last, I thought as I squatted over the latrine. But how wrong could I be? Suddenly a soaking wet mop head was thrust under the space at the base of the door giving my feet a good soaking. Fortunately, the rest of me escaped. This particular cleaner obviously wasn't concerned about any personal feelings. She had a job to do and got on with it regardless.

We headed out of the bus station, turned left into Beijing Lu or Beijing Road, and made our way on foot to the Kun Hu Hotel a short distance away. For incredibly little money we settled on a two-night stay in a room containing three single beds, a small cupboard and a piece of string that stretched from wall to wall that acted as a clothesline. In this establishment, no room keys were given and to gain access to your room you had to track down a miserable room maid who, with a deep sigh, would unlock the door when it was convenient for her. The facilities were basic but adequate. Vicky and I showered in a grey concrete, windowless room which was the communal bathroom for the ladies. Ian went off to the men's unit. After completion of our ablutions the three of us stood in a small space with a tap mounted above a large concrete slab and washed our smalls with a bar of soap and spread them out to dry on the line in our room.

Chapter 15

"It's going to be filter coffee and crispy bread rolls for our breakfast this morning. We know of a little café in the old French quarter," said Vicky. "It's a favourite of ours, and we're sure you'll love it too."

On the way, I could have spent hours in the small brightly lit shops that lined Beijing Lu. I loved loitering and buying all the little things I was unable to find locally: items like a nailbrush and a nail file that, to me, were vital. They were probably on sale in Xiaguan, but somehow, I could never find them. In the foyers of the big hotels I made a mental note of the branded face creams, deodorants, toilet soaps and shower gels. My skin wasn't marvellous but I was determined to take care of it, and buying nice things was an enjoyable way to feel good.

The road was long and straight with congested traffic moving slowly. In the distance, I could hear the wail of several loud sirens and saw all vehicles pull to the side of the road and stop. I expected an ambulance, fire engine or at least a police patrol car. But no, a convoy of four luxury cars with darkened windows sped by with little flags attached to their wings. I was told the occupants were government officials, probably out on a visit, and I had no reason to question it.

As we ambled along and I could see young men peering anxiously over their shoulders as they crouched over small tables. They were selling pirated compact discs, CDs, and video compact discs or VCDs, a primitive form of digital video discs, and DVDs. My friends told me these men would disappear in a flash if the City Management Officials appeared. I learned these uniformed officers or *Chengguan*, were attempting to flush the illegal traders off the streets. They were not known for their gentle treatment.

On street corners, I saw little groups of white-coated physiotherapists and masseurs treating customers as they sat on chairs on the pavements. These professionals were blind. Their touts stood nearby and attracted clients. On different corners, more white-coated people were waiting with forceps and cotton buds at the ready to clean the dirty ears of passers-by. There was no shortage of customers. For a small fee, I stood on a set of scales and had a public weighing! I was delighted with my 10-kilogram weight loss and decided the local diet was obviously suiting me.

At last we arrived in Jinbi Lu. What a lovely street: rows of ageing little houses of French design washed with a dark yellow paint, and windows almost hidden behind green shutters. At street level well-tended pots of scarlet geraniums, yellow pansies and pink busy-lizzies lined the kerbs. Above our heads the foliage from plane trees provided us with much needed shade and coolness.

Ian smiled and said, "What a lovely smell of filter coffee," but of course I couldn't appreciate it. I could only guess the pull of the aroma as we hurried to a small café where we tucked into our promised breakfast of crispy bread rolls and big mugs of steaming black coffee.

Around the corner the scene changed totally. The houses that lined these narrow roads were wood panelled, with paper-lined carved lattice windows. Most of them had balconies with wooden balustrades. Geraniums and leaves of giant spider plants cascaded down and partially hid the odd songbird in its wire cage. The sun shone through wild grasses that sprouted from tiles on the roofs, giving a halo effect. At ground level, poles held lines of washing that fluttered in the breeze.

Along the roadside, little ladies in blue sold fresh vegetables. They weighed them on a set of brass scales with poles that slid along, working on the principle of balance I supposed. Alongside their scales joints of meat were hooked to rails, and featherless ducks were hanging by their necks from low beams. I was taken aback by the steam and smoke that rose from a noodle-making store. I stopped to watch and saw prodigious amounts of sweat drip from workers as they mixed dough with long wooden paddles in huge vats made of wood. Hanging from long rails in front of them were lines of freshly made noodles drying in the sun. So much was happening in this small area I could have stayed all day and watched the busy life going on all around me, but there wasn't time on this visit.

A few streets away Vicky and Ian took me to the animal and bird market. I could hear these feathery bundles singing their little hearts out before we reached them but when I saw how tightly they were packed into their cages I wondered how they could be so happy. The larger birds sang too, but somehow didn't sound quite so tuneful. Owls, in tiny wire prisons, looked miserable and upset as if they knew their destiny was probably the wok - I didn't know. Around me in glass cages were live snakes of all colours and sizes. There were also live frogs and lizards, and fish swimming in large glass tanks. Large flattened dried lizards were laid out on platters. When I asked about them I was told they would probably be used in some sort of Chinese medicine.

That evening we went to a noodle house for dinner. We joined the scrum and laughed as we fought our way to the counter to buy our meal tickets and then to the other side of the room to collect our food. We found an empty table and sat down. We had to keep our bags on our backs, as the floor was filthy. The café floors were always dirty as people slopped their food and coughed and spat as they slurped and sucked noodles into their mouths. We tried to carry on a conversation above the din but had little success because everyone else was shouting, yelling and burping in unison as they ate. In spite of all the distractions, the noodles were yummy.

On the way back to the hotel, we visited the city square and, tucked away in a little building in a far corner, we found a group of people who were singing and acting out part of a

Chinese Opera. We were made welcome and ushered in to get a good view of both the singers and the dancers. A small part of ancient China was alive and well in a hidden corner of this modern city.

The hotel was noisy. On our floor people kept their room doors open and were shouting across corridors to friends. Others were playing cards, never a quiet pastime in this country. A group of young men were creating a real rumpus as they yelled and clapped their hands during an intricate finger game. As they played they downed round after round of whisky, Bai Jiu, similar to the stuff that nearly removed my tonsils on my arrival in Xiaguan. In our room, the water rumbled and clanked in the pipes as we were drifting off to sleep, and the room-maid decided to hammer on our locked door. She had come to remind us our luggage wasn't safe if the door wasn't secure!

Next morning, we returned to the square where, at one side, a group of old men each had a songbird in a bamboo cage. We discovered the men were comparing their birds' lyrical abilities before they covered the cages with green cloths and took them home. In the main part of the square people were dancing an odd two-step to music supplied by a cassette tape, whilst others performed Tai Chi a short distance away. The elderly were swaying in the morning sun, exercising their arms and legs.

We walked to the thousand-year-old Buddhist Yuan Tong Temple, a must for many pilgrims. It was a quiet, serene place, a mere stone's throw away from the hubbub of the city crowds and traffic. A long path led us to an octagonal pavilion and we were surrounded by displays of flowers so beautiful and colourful that I thought Laura Ashley couldn't have made a better arrangement. The temple was almost encircled by a large pond with numerous small paths and bridges leading the way. Once inside I gazed at the beautiful statue of Shakyamuni Buddha, a gift from the Thai royal family. Everywhere people were chanting and kneeling in prayer. This was indeed a remarkable experience and I found the sincerity humbling.

That evening we decided to try another local dish for our meal. We looked to see what was on offer and in the end settled for 'across-the-bridge noodles', an old-time favourite with a lovely tale attached. It was said that many, many years ago a woman had to carry her husband's food over a bridge to a small island where he was studying. In the winter, the food was always cold when she arrived, so one day she decided to take all the ingredients separately and add them to boiling water on her arrival. We chose a restaurant serving this dish and soon steaming bowls of hot water arrived quickly followed by meat and vegetables which we added and cooked as required. The food was tasty but as always, we were accompanied by the usual loud slurps and coughs and spitting routines, and this time periodically interrupted by beggars, eager to take our money.

On our last morning, we headed for the Tea Rooms at the side of Green Lake. These rooms were small partitioned areas on the roofs of houses, where for a small price you could enjoy a pot of tea of your choice and listen to the local storytellers who mesmerised their audiences. As we left we passed half a dozen men who were gambling on the walkway. They played with cards and small crowds had gathered round, some hoping to win a fortune no doubt! Next to them small groups of young Yi ethnic minority boys were painting colourful pictures on squares of paper and selling them to tourists. Scruffy, snotty-nosed kids hung around begging for money while their parents stood watching a short distance away. Then, without warning the *Chengguan* or City Management Officials, arrived and, in what seemed no more than a second, the street was empty, until hordes of primary school children burst from the school gates nearby. They were identically dressed in grey tracksuits and yellow neckties, each one grinning and yelling "ello" at us. Eventually we had to return to our hotel, but not before we gave a few Yuan to a grimy young woman who was rummaging through bins. She would at least have a meal that night.

Our final calls were to stock up supplies of goodies. First, we visited a supermarket to buy half a dozen packets of scrumptious Oreo chocolate biscuits, then around the corner to the Holiday Inn where fresh supplies of delicious cheddar cheese and butter could be obtained from the dining area and taken back to Xiaguan on the bus.

The few days spent together were over far too soon and in the evening, we were on the night bus, heading back to Xiaguan. I felt invigorated and ready to continue my life in China. I had thoroughly enjoyed the company of my new friends, and the break had been rewarding. I had learned so much about this fascinating city and could hardly wait to return.

Chapter 16

I dreamed of getting a computer for planning and writing my lectures, and for emailing my family and friends. I couldn't afford one and it didn't look as if the hospital leaders were going to help me, so I still had to spend many hours hand writing lectures. I tried to keep at least two weeks ahead with my talks, just in case anything untoward should happen to either Rumei or me. And I needed to be sure that my translator understood everything; she was after all an English teacher who had known nothing about nursing till she met me. I was always relieved when, at the end of the day, I could relax and play football with the children or walk up the mountain a short way. The view of the lake was stunning from a height, and if the skies were blue the water was even more blue and tempting. In the evenings Yang Kaishun, my doctor friend, was good company and an hour or so spent helping him with his English was associated with numerous cups of green tea and sharing of amusing anecdotes. Rumei and her parents continued to play an important role in my life and I visited them regularly. Vicky and Ian were also helping me to integrate into the community by introducing me to their friends. Most weeks we would play a serious game of scrabble when we met in Dali, which kept our wits about us. We cooked for each other once a week, producing wonderful meals in our individual kitchens, and caught up on current events.

At the weekends, I would invariably take the bus to Dali and relax for a couple of hours. I would swap books in Jack's Café and enjoy a plate of egg and chips with him and Stella. Sometimes Jack's parents would join us and I would learn more of local life. Now and again I would meet western travellers and it would be good to catch up on recent world news. On one occasion, I met a young man named Zhang Jianbuo. He was leaning against the bar, chatting to Stella. He was handsome, had soft dark eyes and a broad smile. He introduced himself in broken English before breaking off in a giggle, embarrassed at his efforts.

"Peggy, this is my friend Jianbuo." Jack shouted from the kitchen area. "He doesn't speak much English but we went to school together and we don't have many secrets. He's a doctor at the Number Two Peoples' Hospital around the corner. I'm preparing a meal. Will you join us?" he asked as he came into view. "Langer will be coming soon as well. He's another good mate and he works in tourism. He's a good guy for you to meet. He speaks great English and knows the history of all the interesting places to visit."

The five of us sat around the table and talked of many things. Little did I realise at that time that Dr Zhang Jianbuo, or Jianbuo as he became, was to become such an important and respected member of the local community.

Back at the hospital I was getting to know the nurses and learning something of their personalities. There were the keen ones, those eager to learn something new and contribute towards the proceedings and then there were those who were bored and took little interest. They hadn't all wanted to be on a course but had no choice. I enjoyed these group meetings immensely and the greatest challenge for me, and Rumei of course, was to keep the sessions interesting and retain the attention of as many of the students as possible.

The hospital was still nowhere near completion and no one, it seemed, had any idea when it would open. I kept myself occupied and was determined to get out and about as much as possible with Vicky and Ian before they left for Australia. Their local knowledge was outstanding and I wanted to take full advantage of it.

My dragon lady, the head nurse, continually lurked in the background and whenever I felt she was tightening her grip on me, I would confide in Vicky and Ian. This was an enormous relief, and if I thought I had a problem my friends usually had an even bigger one in the shape of their head of their department. The Australians were being hounded, obstructed and criticised for their efforts and this was soul destroying. A few swigs of the Chinese Brandy and a good talk usually dried the tears and cured the problems, for a short while anyway. We decided that we would not be beaten and perhaps it was part of the work remit for all foreigners to have a 'dragon' in one form or another.

"On Saturday, we'll go to Xizhou," said Vicky. "It's an interesting Bai Village on the side of the lake and it's where Bryan and Silvia live with their children, Jamie and Miranda. I think you met Bryan a few weeks ago when he paid you a visit. Anyway, we have to go to Dali then catch a mini-bus. It'll take nearly two hours to get there, so we'll have to make a fairly early start. We'll take some of that cheese and butter we bought in Kunming. It's something we always do for each other and it's a nice little treat".

The day came and, as we approached the village of Xizhou, we drove by the pretty Wanhua Brook with its thickets of tall, swaying bamboos and willows. At the terminus people seemed to be hurrying in every direction. Some poorly dressed men with thin scrawny horses harnessed to homemade carriages, shouted and beckoned to us. They hoped to give us a ride to the hotel, but we wanted to walk the short distance to our friend's house.

The majority of the women we passed on the way wore their colourful Bai outfits. Many were carrying large wicker baskets on their backs. Their bodies were bent as they struggled with heavy loads of fresh fruit and vegetables. We followed the crowd and almost immediately came across a bazaar in a large cobbled square. Water ran around the large pebbles as the produce was hosed and sprinkled to keep its freshness and the same dirty water trickled between our toes.

"There are some wonderful smells here." said Ian. "The fruit and veggies are so fresh and the herbs are so heady. It's a pity you can't appreciate it. Unfortunately, it's also mixed with the smell of horse manure and unwashed bodies! But, even so, this is rural China and I'm sorry you miss so much of it".

We slowly made our way towards a narrow street with shops that overflowed with goods. Toys and clothes spilled onto the road and partially hid the little ladies who sat on low stools embroidering colourful camellia flowers on to black velvet cloth. Narrow alleyways that led to homes went off in all directions; some were concreted but most were compressed soil. In one area, we watched as two women were winnowing. They separated the chaff from the grain with long flails that seemed to twist as they were swung high into the air before being crashed down on the corn. The women stopped now and again to sift the chaff from the seed using large homemade willow sieves. Carefully they put the grain into hessian sacks.

The road led into the town square, where little old ladies sat in little groups and drank green tea and ate steamed paus, little cakes similar to sweet buns. The old men sat across the area in noisy gangs, smoking cigarettes and playing Chinese Chess, a tactical game for two players. It's similar to our Chess but represents a battle between two armies with the aim of capturing the enemy's king.

We passed the only hotel with its unkempt gardens and lines of snow-white sheets blowing in the breeze. We walked along muddy paths, over small streams and eventually came to Bryan and Silvia's house, which was surrounded by a high brick wall and protected by large metal gates. We spent a pleasant couple of hours playing with Jamie, who was five and Miranda, just three. This couple had been in China for several years and were studying for PhDs in some kind of applied linguistics. Their house was filled with laughter and happiness and it became something of a home away from home. There was always a welcome and it was somewhere to relax, be myself and have a good chat. The kids were amazing because, like their parents, they could speak in four languages - English, Italian, Chinese and the local Bai tongue. It was reassuring to have such a hospitable couple living so near and I happily accepted the offer to visit whenever I could.

As he walked with us to the bus stop to make our journey home, Bryan gave me a potted history of the village. Back in the 10th century, he said, Xizhou had been a military fortress during the reign of the Nanzhao Kingdom, but had then developed into an important commercial centre. In 1949, when Chairman Mao came to power, the half dozen wealthy landowners who lived and controlled the area were ousted and dispersed by the Red Army. Peasants replaced these families, with sometimes six or seven families living in each grand house. Nowadays it is a busy commuting centre, with people travelling to various cities including Dali, Xiaguan, Kunming and way beyond.

I'd fallen in love with Xizhou and looked forward to my next visit.

Chapter 17

I loved my teaching role and, although this job was nothing like the original remit of improving the inpatient care at the new Affiliated Hospital I'd originally accepted from VSO, I was adaptable and felt I was making a difference, no matter how small. My Royal Marsden Manual of Clinical Nursing had been thoroughly studied and used and was beginning to look tired, dog-eared and decidedly scruffy. Initially I was told the Nursing Practical Room would be at my disposal for demonstrations, but this was not to be, like so many other broken promises. I never actually saw this facility and I wondered if indeed it did exist. But, in spite of all the problems, my teaching sessions were pleasurable and I looked forward to them. I knew they would come to an end when the term ended and as the hospital was nowhere near completion I worried that I might be made redundant. Did I want repatriation? At the end of the day there might not be a choice.

"Are you ready?" Rumei shouted as she arrived at my apartment. "Have you remembered the end of term party with the nurses? We are going on a boat to Jin Soa Island in the middle of lake. Make sure you wear your trainers because we'll be doing some walking."

I was so glad Rumei had been invited. She would be the vital link between us all, ensuring there would be no communication problems. We set off together and when we met the nurses we found several English-speaking doctors had decided to join us. Everyone was looking forward to a fun day out.

Our boat was one of many moored alongside the lake frontage. Some were small, while others were huge, taking upwards of five hundred passengers. Ours was tiny by comparison and could accommodate maybe fifty. Once on board my mind drifted towards the safety aspect. I looked around for lifebelts, but there were none and I felt more than a little concerned when the engine throbbed into life. As we left our mooring nobody showed any emotion. Was I alone in my unease? Was I being stupid? There was nothing I could do; a lone query wouldn't alter the situation so I decided to make the best of things and put on a brave face. I soon came to the conclusion that the lack of any lifesaving equipment was normal practice and had to be accepted.

"Jin Soa Island is a popular place for visitors." Rumei said. "It's small and shaped a bit like a peanut. We'll have plenty of time to walk around and I know you'll love it. We'll meet some of the fishermen and their families who live there all year round. They go shopping in Xiaguan when they need something special, but they are more or less self-sufficient. Their children go to school in Xiaguan and stay as boarders."

As we headed away from the anchorage, the scenery was extraordinary. Hazy-purple coloured mountains almost surrounded the lake. The water reflected the colour of the sky and was a deep blue, but at times it became quite green as the submerged stems of the reeds almost broke the surface. This stretch of water was approximately forty kilometres long and twenty kilometres wide and sported an abundance of fish. Four aging wooden junks with torn and tatty sails looked romantic and majestic as they glided by. The enormity of their huge bulks was belittled by the modest sound of their sails flapping in the wind. We passed small, canopied, metal fishing boats with two or three people on board using a conical scoop net on a triangular metal frame. This was thrown into the water and hauled back to reveal the catch. It was a lovely journey and a breath-taking introduction to the joys of sailing on the lake.

It took an hour or so to reach the island and, as we anchored a young man brought a bucketful of small live fish on board. Two girls followed him, one with a huge pot of rice and some chilli peppers and the other with a pile of bowls and chopsticks. My colleagues lit a portable gas heater and, after a wok and a bottle of oil had been produced, the cooking began. I have never cared much for fish and felt a little troubled, but I wasn't alone because the fish didn't like it much either. They kept trying to jump out of the wok, only to be thrown back into the smoking oil if they made it as far as the bench or the floor in their struggle for freedom.

The meal began and whole fish were gobbled down. I copied my friends and quickly discovered that you spat out the bits you didn't want and nobody seemed to notice the large pile of heads, tails and bones around my feet. The rice was washed down with a welcome Dali Beer.

A walk around the island revealed a number of small white- painted stone cottages which were the homes of local fishermen. Groups of men were sitting in the sunshine folding nets. They stopped to give us a wave and a smile. Others were sitting at low tables playing noisy card games. Their women folk were making and mending nets, and as a side-line made pretty little shell souvenirs for visitors. They seemed content with their lives and looked well.

On the shoreline, the water was warm and clear but stony underfoot and a few brave souls paddled. The men rolled their trouser legs up and the women, almost hidden under hats and umbrellas, tucked their skirts into their knicker legs or rolled up their trouser legs too. I was transported back to the 1920's, when pictures showed similar sights on English beaches. I had a little giggle, took a photo and continued on my way. As the sun began to sink behind the mountains we slowly made our way back to the boat. We'd had a great day and I'd really enjoyed my first outing on the lake, with or without lifebelts.

Meanwhile, back at the hospital a message was waiting for me to prepare an end of term examination for the students. My interpreter and I had been working together for more than three months and had covered most of the topics the nurses had requested at the start of the term. These women had become inquisitive and the debates that followed my talks were noisy and satisfying and I had certainly learned a great deal from them.

I worked on a test paper that included a questionnaire to evaluate my ability, not only in working with a translator but also how well we had functioned as a team. Rumei and I were delighted with the results. The nurses felt we had been very successful working together and were sorry to lose us. They all passed the examination with flying colours and I sent a report echoing their sentiments to the VSO office in Beijing.

The term was drawing to a close and I was at a loss to know what to do. My employment in the hospital was about to end just as I had begun to enjoy my new surroundings. I didn't particularly want to go back to England. I missed my home, family and friends enormously, but felt I was coping with my new life. The Guardian Monthly had kept me more or less up to date with world affairs, but it took six weeks to arrive and had been well censored before it reached me. Often whole sections had been cut out and sometimes the whole paper was confiscated. The varied assortment of glossy magazines sent faithfully every month by Dorothy, a wonderful sister-in-law from my first marriage, provided me with easy reading and was a real link with home. These magazines also gave my Chinese friends a great insight to life in the West as they read articles, studied the fashions and gazed at some of the way-out hairstyles. Their shyness disappeared as I gave answers to their never-ending questions.

Then my thoughts turned to what about my own hair? I'd been in Xiaguan for three months and really needed a trim as my hair was long and unruly. But where should I go? I didn't know. In a country where almost every single person has black hair and it's either long, in a pony-tail or in something that resembled a 'pudding basin' style I knew I would have a problem. And the more I thought about it, the worse it became. China is not known for its ethnic diversity and as I didn't resemble anything remotely native there were times when I felt something akin to being a freak. This might happen when complete strangers approached to touch my hair, face or arms simply because I was pale and surely interesting. My brown hair had blond highlights. It was different and was untidy. I knew I would have to take the plunge and visit a hairdresser, and judging by the way I looked it would have to be sooner rather than later. So, the day came when I found enough courage to visit what I assumed to be a fairly up-market salon in Dali. I reckoned the staff had seen western tourists and perhaps had even styled some of their hair.

The two hairdressers were busy and as I waited my turn I grew anxious. I couldn't speak enough of the language to tell them exactly what I wanted and there were no style magazines. It wasn't long before the girls came to me. They were in deep discussion as they ran their fingers through my tresses. Then, my head was gently pushed into an enamel bowl and warm water started to run through my locks. I was lulled into a false sense of security and began to feel at ease. After a quick towel dry the scissors went into action and in ten minutes flat I emerged into the sunshine with my new 'pudding basin' style.

As for the hairdressers, had they tried to make me one of them? But I was in China and these girls had done their best and they knew no other way! There was little opportunity to step from the straight and narrow road I was travelling on. I hadn't thought that this would include my hair-style.

Eventually I found a girl who, with a razor in her hand, did a much better job and gave me a style of some kind. I stayed with her for the rest of my placement.

One thing for sure, every day was special and life was never a bore.

I'd been away for months, phone calls home to family and friends in England were expensive, so were few and far between. It was easy to detect that a third person was always listening-in to my calls but it didn't worry me. I just hoped they enjoyed the conversations and thought perhaps their spoken English might improve. But more than that, I was living in one of the most beautiful parts of China and wanted to know so much more.

I contacted the VSO head office in Beijing and with their consent I ventured into the Medical College some three kilometres away and met with David and Charles from the Foreign Affairs Department to discuss the problem of the non-completion of the Affiliated Hospital. I was delighted to be offered a new role as teacher of British Nursing Practises to Chinese medical personnel and help them with their English. This was to begin at the start of the next term and I would be provided with a flat within the campus grounds at the college.

Unfortunately, I would lose my interpreter. The doctors had all learnt English at school and had some understanding of the language but needed help with the spoken word. I would also be given the opportunity to work alongside some nurses at a nearby clinic.

That evening Vicky, Ian and I discussed my new job at length and we felt that although I wasn't qualified to teach English as a foreign language, I did possess a teaching diploma in nursing and had already proved my ability with the nurses. I felt that this role was well within my capability and decided to go for it. The three of us also made plans for a holiday in Guizhou, the neighbouring Province, early in the summer prior to their return to Australia, as their placement had come to an end.

I knew I would miss these two people terribly when they left China. Without the brilliant friendship and support they gave in my early days I knew I wouldn't have managed as well as I did. But I had survived and knew that life would go on. I felt confident with my new situation and would be able to say goodbye to my dragon head nurse, well almost, when I moved to my new premises in September 1997.

Chapter 18

My first sight of Chong'an, a small village in the Province of Guizhou, took place one evening following a nightmare bus ride from Kaili. In fact, almost the whole journey had been a painful one for me because I had bruised my bum.

The trip had been carefully planned: a night bus from Dali to Kunming, train from Kunming to Kaili in Guizhou Province, then local bus to our final destination of Chong'an, inhabited mainly by Miao, Gezia and Dong ethnic minority groups. My guide book said it was a pretty place with seven bridges that spanned a river.

The three of us were in high spirits as we boarded the night bus from Dali to Kunming Railway Station on the first leg of our trip early in July. Once there we joined the crowds and eventually bought our tickets for hard sleepers for the train journey to Kaili. We had a choice of expensive soft comfortable sleeper bunks, hard sleeper bunks, hard seats or standing room. We had a thirty-six-hour trip ahead of us and settled for the cheaper, but bearable hard bunks. A female official escorted us to an upstairs waiting room at the station that was reserved for foreigners only. She would return and lead us to our compartment when the train arrived. We drank green tea as the rain lashed down, grateful for the fact that we were at least dry, unlike the crowds of Chinese who stood and looked miserable as they huddled under umbrellas in the area around the station.

Exactly on time the train pulled in and our guide arrived to escort us to the platform. Half way down the long, wet metal staircase I tripped and slithered and bumped my way down, making a grand entrance on to the rain sodden platform. People seemed to appear from all directions to help me to my feet. I stood for a few moments, took a deep breath, realised I was still in one piece and slowly made my way to the waiting train. I had my rucksack on my back and fortunately this had taken the brunt of the fall, which only left me with a bruised backside and somewhat shaken. This holiday was important. The three of us had looked forward to exploring a new place and I wasn't about to let my friends, or myself, down if I could help it.

We were led to our booked bunks, which were in a small compartment containing six berths, three on each side and stacked one above the other. They were a bit like the hard couches you find in doctors' waiting rooms. The bottom bed was always the favourite because the centre one was too shallow to allow one to sit up, but was fine for sleeping. The top bunk was shallow as well, but had the added bonus of a constant blast from the air-conditioning system! Fortunately, Vicky had booked the two bottom bunks and one of the middle ones, so we were fairly comfortable. By day all the passengers used the bottom bunks for sitting on and at night climbed the ladders and settled down in separate beds: well, for most of the time.

Our guide exchanged our tickets for metal tags and assured us that we would be informed when we reached our destination. We secured our bags to the metal luggage racks with our bike chains and padlocks and settled down, with me lying on my front to take the pressure off my painful bruised bum.

We sped past paddy fields, forests and lakes, and small towns, with periodic stops at stations where, through the open windows, we bought noodles, rice and steamed bread from vendors on the platforms. Mega-size flasks of boiling water were replaced regularly in the compartment, which made tea and coffee making a simple and cheap affair. A visit to the toilet was interesting to say the least. There was a hole in the floor of a cubicle with no door and as you squatted blasts of chilly air would rush up and hit you. It was quite a strange sensation but as always, I was prepared to try anything at least once, or twice; or more if absolutely necessary! We rested, enjoyed each other's company and sometimes chatted to our fellow companions. The time flew by.

Kaili was a tiny town but it was also the gateway to several ethnic minority groups in the south-eastern area of Guizhou Province. We had an overnight stop there. Little English was spoken; in fact, we didn't see any other foreigners, so at that time visitors were probably few and far between. We strolled through the almost deserted streets and, by sheer chance, came across a pharmacy where I bought some cooling dressings to put on my bruises later in the day. We booked a three-bedded room for one night at the Petroleum Hotel, the only establishment where foreigners could stay. The reception area was dusty and dirty, but it did boast a huge brass plate which proudly stated that tourists were welcome as the place was registered to accept aliens. Our large room contained three single beds and was shabby and none too clean. Large spider webs hung from the ceiling and formed black lacy patterns on the walls, and the carpet between our beds was covered in coffee stains and cigarette burns. But the sheets were fresh and crisp and in spite of our surroundings we slept well that night.

Next morning, we boarded the battered bus to Chong'an. It would take over an hour to reach our destination and we hoped the vehicle would make it. Our driver tripped and fell up the steps as he entered the crowded vehicle. His glasses had lenses like the bottoms of Coke bottles and we did wonder if he could see at all. He started the engine and we set off. All went well till we came to some road works a short distance away when, instead of veering away from the partly prepared new surface, he ploughed straight into it and the bus came to a grinding halt. Chaos broke out amongst the passengers and the driver was replaced by a younger man who drove like a madman. The edges of the roads were also the edges of steep ravines, and there were no crash barriers. When going around tight bends the driver honked his horn continuously to alert oncoming vehicles but never seemed to slow down, consequently there was much handrail gripping and grimacing among the passengers, including me. Thankfully, we drew up at our destination quite safely.

Five lazy, hazy days were spent in Chong'an. Such a picturesque riverside village with its little wooden houses, endless rice terraces and hardworking peasants who wore huge cone-shaped straw hats as they guided their slow-plodding buffaloes along dirt paths. We spent hours at the market, which occurred every fifth day and gazed at goods brought down from the mountains to be sold. You could buy literally anything, ranging from brightly embroidered clothes and hand-made furniture to farm tools and livestock. It was quite a sight and an almost overwhelming experience. In the evenings, the cicadas serenaded us with their unique variable shrilling sounds, quiet at first before reaching an almost deafening crescendo. Huge black butterflies settled on the flowers that sat in small pots in the guesthouse gardens and the air was still.

Many of the women and girls looked as if they had goitres, or enlarged thyroid glands, and most had bruise marks on their necks caused by moxabustion, when heat from the burning of the herb moxa was applied to the acupuncture points. This was the local cure for an obvious iodine deficiency. But all the girls were pretty, particularly those from the Gezia, a branch of the Miao ethnic minority tribe. They wore embroidered skullcaps and navy crossover tops over black trousers. The married women wore the same outfits, but had white patterned hats, which flared out at their ears. Coloured strings topped their bonnets.

An idyllic day was spent cruising up and down the beautiful river in a long boat with a single boatman, a noisy engine and a couple of oars. We sailed lazily along, enjoying solitude when the engine was silenced. We listened to the songs of birds accompanied by sounds of contented buffaloes as they wallowed in deeper waters. On the banks, women washed clothes using the tried and tested method of rubbing soap on the garments before dashing them against the rocks. Such hard work, but these people were laughing and chatting together, making the task more bearable.

I never did see the bridges, but to me this whole area was yet another of China's hidden treasures. Wearily we returned to our accommodation and were lulled to sleep by the lilting sounds of a peasant girl as she sang a beautiful love song at the water's edge.

On reflection, I could see these few days had provided me with a good insight into the lives of ordinary people, individuals who had little or nothing, but seemed in many ways to be happier and more content than the wealthy folk I'd come across. The hospitality they offered was almost beyond anything I'd experienced. Their expectations didn't seem to extend much beyond acquiring an education for their children, thus ensuring them a better life.

Chapter 19

I have a small Jade Buddha that hangs from a length of finely plaited red cord attached to the rear-view mirror of my car. It was a gift from Wu Ling and I carry it everywhere in the belief that I will be safe. Wu Ling was a twenty-six-year-old English teacher at the Number Two Middle School in Dali. She was an attractive, quiet little soul who dreamed of travelling the world. Quite an ambition for one who lived what appeared to me such a dull life in a miserable little bed-sit containing no more than a single bed, a table and two chairs. The antiquated cooking, washing and toilet facilities were shared with the many others who lived and worked within the two thousand pupil complex. Life was hard, but she had no choice. The few possessions that this teacher owned were stored in a box under her bed. The grey concrete walls inside her space were adorned with the odd picture or magazine cuttings. The wire that held the faded curtain around her bed acted as a hanging place for her few clothes. Her family lived in Kunming and the journey to Dali was the greatest distance she had ever travelled.

Most of her free time was spent marking papers or preparing lessons at the table in her room. Sometimes she read English classics. My glossy western magazines gave her a lot of pleasure and we chatted and gazed for hours at the Western fashions and commercial goodies. She loved romantic stories, but the holiday features fascinated her most. Deep down she was strong and I admired her spirit. Bit by bit our friendship grew and we made plans for a trip together in August after I had returned from Chong' An. We would visit Lijiang and Zhongdian to the north of Dali, but still within Yunnan Province.

It was a beautiful day as a smiling Wu Ling met me in Dali for breakfast at the start of our adventure. The peace was suddenly shattered by raised voices; an argument had broken out at the bus ticket booth. A young Japanese man was leaning against the booth looking puzzled. He wanted to go to Lijiang but had been refused a ticket for some reason. I sympathised and knew exactly how frustrated he felt and after talking to my friend a decision was made that he could travel with us, at least for the first part of our journey. As I approached the man, whose name was Toshi, his face broke into a huge grin and he shouted, "Yes. Yes. I'd love to come with you." I bought three tickets for the local bus with no fuss.

The drive to Lijiang took six hours and was spectacular. The land running alongside the lake was green with vegetables and as we drove past we could see small plots of rice being harvested with scythes and tied into sheaves. Near the roadway were huge pools where lotus plants spread their leaves on the surface, and fish caused little ripples in the sunlight as their snouts broke the surface to gulp air. Peasants in cone shaped hats were everywhere, some hoeing and others mixing and spreading compost made from night soil, brought in overflowing honey buckets from the local latrines.

A few kilometres out of town we passed a lone Buddhist temple built into the mountainside, and in the distance, we could see people slowly making their way towards it. Groups of girls and boys were cycling home from school with their books in identical packs on their backs. Some of the men and women physically hauled handcarts laden with mountains of cabbages and sheaves of rice straw. We drove alongside horse-drawn carts with passengers returning from town, their plastic bags filled with produce balanced on their knees. Many people just walked along the roadside carrying their hoes on their shoulders. As we approached the north end of the lake, a huge cement factory built into the beautiful mountainside belched pollution into the atmosphere and small clay ovens near the edge of the highway competed to intensify the smoke-laden air.

We bounced along in our old mini bus over surfaces that were sometimes metalled, but often cobbled. The seats were unbelievably uncomfortable as we followed the narrow asphalt strip as it snaked up the mountain and cut through fields of cotton trees, sugar cane and sorghum. We travelled through pine forests that led to mountain passes then down to lush, green valleys. We followed rivers and streams where people washed their clothes, their vegetables and their joints of meat, while the buffaloes wallowed nearby. Lining the roads were numerous tiny untidy villages where small, grimy people manufactured tiles in clouds of dust, while their tethered buffaloes, blindfolded and dusty, trudged round and round to mix the moist clay.

Occasionally we caught glimpses of tall white Pagodas, which stood proudly on high as if watching over the people and the countryside below. As we drew nearer Lijiang, the Jade Dragon Snow Mountain with its snow-covered peaks towered over the city like a magnificent halo.

It was getting dark when we arrived and we hadn't booked any rooms. We didn't have much money between us and wondered if we could afford, or indeed find anywhere to sleep. It seemed almost everyone had come to town, filling all the hotels and guesthouses, because we had arrived in the middle of the Torch Festival. This traditional holiday was celebrated by the Yi ethnic minority people whose aim was to rid the crops of the greedy legendary insects which ate everything in sight and, according to local superstition, blazing torches had to be burned for three days and nights, accompanied by loud singing and dancing. As darkness fell our accommodation problem grew worse. Wu Ling could stay with Toshi and me in a hotel or guesthouse authorised to accept foreigners, if the management approved of her documents. Toshi and I could not officially stay in a Chinese only establishment. We trudged around for what seemed like hours until finally Wu Ling persuaded the landlord of a Chinese-only hotel to accept us using her identity card and money offered by Toshi and me as a bribe. The only available room contained three single beds. It was that or a night under the stars on rice straw mats. Under the circumstances that might have been the better option because our room was filthy, with the floor covered in drink stains and cigarette ends. At the end of a corridor an indescribable communal latrine stood next to equally bad shower facilities. The whole outfit was ghastly; nevertheless, our accommodation was secured and we sat over a meal of noodle soup, taking part in the celebrations until the early hours. Our hosts made music with wind instruments fashioned from bamboo. The Yi girls were striking. Their eye-catching outfits of large square brimmed hats, lined with red cloth and edged with braid, together with side-fastening colourful blouses over multi-coloured skirts, made them attract attention as they sang. They danced and flared their torches, not only from the rooftops but around us as well. Firecrackers were exploding in every direction and everyone was in high spirits.

We sat and chatted as we watched the party. Toshi told us he was twenty-five years old and had just graduated from University. He decided to have a gap year and travel the world with China being his first port of call. When he returned to Japan he would join the family engineering business and possibly never benefit from another holiday till he retired, such was his accepted way of life. Wu Ling chatted about her travel aspirations and I told them both about my life in England. When it came to bedding down for the night I felt quite sorry for Wu Ling. She had lived a very sheltered life and had never been in such close contact with a man before, let alone slept in the same room. But Toshi was a perfect gentleman and I told her to pretend that he wasn't there. She knew that I would look after her anyway. We didn't undress and as we settled down for a few hours' sleep and I have an unforgettable memory of Toshi as he gingerly sniffed the duvet and pillow.

"This whole place stinks. It's terrible. It's more than that. It's very terrible," he said, as he closed his eyes.

And he was so right. My eyes told me more than I needed to know and I knew I'd escaped many of the less appealing realities of beautiful rural China, until now.

In the morning, after numerous cups of green tea made with the usual supply of boiled water, we made our way to the showers. The sexes were separated and Wu Ling and I stood naked under blasts of cold water, which ran straight from a row of pipes fixed to the ceiling. There were no curtains for privacy and no showerheads to reduce the force of the water, but the dousing was invigorating and it felt good to be clean again and have a change of clothing. Toshi had had a similar experience with his ablutions and we laughed together as we packed our dirty clothes into tightly knotted plastic bags and relived the previous night's events.

We headed towards the old town for breakfast. Even though extensive damage was still visible from an earthquake in 1996, the town was an enchanting jumble of old rickety wooden buildings, little bridges that crossed a maze of canals and rivers, and narrow cobbled passageways that seemed to lead off in every direction. We chose a pretty little café on the banks of a canal and watched the world go by as we tucked into the local speciality of griddlecakes and chatted to the locals.

Lijiang is traditionally the home of another ethnic minority group, the Naxi people. The older women wear dark blue caps and black or blue aprons over blue blouses and black trousers. A black cape with a white lining and front cross over straps completes the outfit. This not only prevents chafing from the heavy baskets they carry on their backs but also depicts the heavens, with seven circles denoting stars embroidered on the back. We soaked up the tranquil atmosphere while discussing our next move. We had been included and taken part in the local festive activities and it had been a sheer delight to watch the different ethnic groups enjoy each other's company in such congenial surroundings. They had all made us so welcome but the truth was we didn't relish the thought of another night in that dirty hotel and we decided to head up north to Zhongdian. This town, sometimes known as Shangri La, is in Deqing Prefecture in the north of Yunnan Province. We decided to explore more of Lijiang on our return journey. Again, it wasn't possible to make an advanced room booking at our new destination of Zhongdian, but we were full of hope and decided to take potluck.

With full stomachs, we heaved our rucksacks onto our backs and slowly made our way back to the bus station on the edge of the new part of the town. The previous night's celebrations had left rubbish strewn everywhere and the spent ribbons of firecrackers looked like red confetti as bundles of it lay on the walkways. On some rooftops, the half-burnt remains of huge torches hung precariously from the eaves, and all around us groups were still in party mood as they sang and danced and made their way to their various destinations.

The station itself was orderly with rows of buses, both ancient and modern. The waiting area contained a mass of noisy humanity that stood in ragged bunches near the ticketing office. I joined other travellers in a long line which one could only laughingly refer to as a queue, and managed to buy our three tickets for the bus. By now I had learned that a loaded bag on my back was a good weapon; it enabled me to keep my place in the disorderly file and allowed me to push and shove as good as, if not better than, the next person.

It was an hour before our bus was due to leave so we squatted on our bags and took in the local life. Peddlers sold an assortment of snacks and seemed to be in every corner or tiny space. It wasn't long before we decided to indulge ourselves. There were short twisted lengths of deep fried rice, little rolls of steamed bread and a type of pancake made from crushed maize and milk. This was produced by dipping one ladle into the mixture, then placing another one on the top and submerging the lot into a vat of a smoking hot liquid that resembled engine oil. It cooked in seconds and the result was as delicious a wafer-type snack as I have ever tasted. I had long since decided that, as far as street food was concerned, if I could actually see the water boiling, or if smoke rose from the oil, few bugs would be able to survive. It was also important to see the food being cooked. That philosophy held me in good stead for the whole of my stay in South East Asia.

The bus pulled in and everyone scrambled to get on board. As usual Wu Ling, Toshi and I waited patiently. Our seats were numbered and no way would the driver let anyone else take our places that we had booked and paid for. Occasionally Japanese travellers were not treated kindly in China, as we had seen in Dali, so we pretended Toshi was Chinese. Obviously, his features were different, but there were so many ethnic minority people in the area that nobody took much notice. He had to keep quiet and let Wu Ling do the talking.

The driver welcomed us on board with a big smile enhanced by the loss of two front teeth. The vehicle was a normal sized single-decker and in no time every seat was occupied. In the front, a small group of extra passengers stood in the stairwell. Immediately behind the driver three live chickens sat silently on the axle housing with their feet tied together. An old man in his blue Mao suit found a few spare inches beside them. The gangway was piled high as usual with all sorts of stuff, ranging from cardboard boxes to small farm implements, making it impossible to beat a hasty retreat should the need arise. We stowed our bags in the overhead compartments and sat down.

The highway headed north and soon we ran out of civilisation and metalled road. As before, the sound of sunflower seed husks being separated and spat onto the floor was constant, followed by the noisy chewing of kernels was accompanied by the continual click of cigarette lighters. The inevitable round of hawking, coughing and spitting followed these events. Toshi screwed his nose up and commented on the body odour, which was made worse by the heat and the closeness of the other passengers. Wedged tightly into our seats we bumped our way along past deep, wooded gorges with nothing that remotely resembled a crash barrier to prevent the bus from plunging into the ravines. From time to time we stopped to let people get off in remote places and I wondered how far they had to walk along the mud tracks to their homes.

Our old banger made slow, grinding progress up the mountains giving us ample time to absorb the beautiful views of snow covered peaks and green valleys. We had a comfort and refreshment stop at a tiny café that stood all alone on a steep mountain slope. I was very glad to find a hosepipe trailing out from the café, as my hands needed a good wash before venturing inside for a delicious bowl of noodle soup. It was strange how quickly I became used to a totally different diet in such a short space of time; my survival instincts had certainly kicked in!

Soon we were on our way once more. We were excited at the idea of spending a few days in Zhongdian, a town almost on the Tibetan border, and we had no idea what to expect. The bus trundled on until eventually we descended to an almost level, lush, grassy plain bounded by pine-forested mountains. Tiny villages with huge wooden drying racks, which looked like giants' armchairs, were dotted at intervals. Herds of yak, with their long black and white coats blowing in the breeze, were scattered in little groups on the wide grassy areas. Some ponies galloped around in circles while others left their grazing to stare at us. We realised we were on the Tibetan Plateau and saw in the distance the town of Zhongdian.

The town stood at some three thousand, five hundred metres above sea level. It was bitterly cold in the winter with snow lasting on the mountain peaks till late April or May. But now it was July and the rains had come and everywhere was green. My handbook told us the majority of the inhabitants were Tibetans and Khamba, a branch of this group, but also included were the Han, Hui or Muslim, Naxi and Bai ethnic people. But whatever ethnic minority group people belonged to, they were all smiles as they welcomed us.

Wide streets were lined with whitewashed three-storey houses. Timbers, which supported these buildings, were painted in many different shades of reds, and with the bright greens of the leafy trees there was a near kaleidoscope effect. People were in little groups and nobody seemed to be in a hurry. Even yak strolled lazily along, stopping now and again for a drink from waterways that ran alongside the lanes. Well-fed horses were tethered outside coffee shops where their Tibetan owners drank black coffee. These tall handsome men with long black hair shining from a Yak butter dressing looked good in their high boots and broad brimmed hats. Silver-studded belts held long knives in elaborate sheaths tightly around their waists. Most of the Tibetan women wore traditional style colourful side-opening embroidered vests over long sleeved white blouses. Short pleated skirts over black trousers and boots completed the outfits. Their hair was long and braided before being coiled around their heads, which were covered with small caps decorated with colourful wools plaited around the edges. Beautiful white even teeth enhanced lovely smiles and pretty faces.

We needed a guesthouse and settled for a slightly more upmarket one this time, again using Wu Ling's identity cards. We took two beds in a twenty-bedded dormitory for females and a single for Toshi in the men's unit. The place was spotless, sheets were clean and Toshi looked happy. In his broken English, he assured me it was okay. Wu Ling and I didn't know anything about the other women, who would share the room, but at least we would be together and there was always safety in numbers.

We ate in a tiny cafe within a large tent and had some delicious ham, fried potatoes, chilli and onions and drank the salty yak-butter tea. The whole feast was washed down with local beer that was cloudy and had grains of barley floating on the surface. We felt mellow as we dawdled back to our guesthouse and looked forward to a good night's sleep, but once there we discovered the toilet and washroom area was under lock and key! Fortunately, there were bushes nearby, always a much better option than most Chinese public toilets.

Next day we wandered into shops stocked with dazzling silver and brass curios, clothes, hand-woven cloths and rolls of cotton material. Others sold solid wooden furniture, wood burning stoves and what seemed to be endless rows of knives with fine carvings on both the handles and the blades. Outside a furniture shop we saw a crowd of people gathered on the pavement surrounding a little boy aged about three years. He was standing in a tall wicker basket. A birthmark on the left side of his face stretched from his ear to his mouth and into his neck. Because of the different skin pigmentation in this part of the world, the birthmark was black rather than the wine-coloured stains I was familiar with. This particular one had long black hairs sprouting from it. The father stood proudly beside his son and accepted money and gifts from passers-by. At that time the whole thing sickened me, but the child and his family looked happy and well fed and I came to the conclusion that in times of extreme poverty, exhibiting a curiosity is acceptable and may even be considered a respectable way for family survival.

Five kilometres north of Zhongdian lay the Buddhist Guiha Monastery, a 300-year-old building on the site of the old Songzhanlin village, home to hundreds of monks. We made this journey on foot, the steep narrow road winding its way through small villages. Again, the houses had three stories, but in this area the animals lived on the ground floor, families on the second with the sleeping arrangement on the third. Colourful rectangular shaped prayer flags attached to poles were leaning out of highly decorated trapezium shaped window frames. These simple devices fluttered in the breeze and seemed to harmonise the environment and increase the general feeling of contentment and wellbeing. On an open area, we saw a large white pagoda surrounded by piles of sacred rocks lined with dozens of simple colourful prayer flags.

A short distance ahead, on the top of a small hill, stood the Guiha Temple. This beautiful sacred building looked so majestic with the peace and quiet broken only by the sounds of four young novices gathering and sawing wood. Brightly coloured frescoes of religious imagery covered the exterior walls of the monastery. Inside, the walls of the main hall were adorned with paintings of Buddha and imaginary beasts, which surrounded golden statues. The colour red dominated everything, from the robes of the monks and novices to the posts, rafters, benches and tables. Embroidered silk banners hung from the rafters and butter lamps, bronze bells and paintings of lamas stood on the altar. We sat and listened to the chanting of scriptures, totally engrossed in our surroundings and I wished I could smell the incense that burned all round us in ornate little butter lamps.

Deep in thought the three of us wandered around the grounds. We turned the large brightly painted prayer wheels, always in a clockwise direction. The spiritual atmosphere made me feel calm. I think it had the same effect on Toshi and Wu Ling because we ambled back to Zhongdian in almost total silence.

We loved the little town and had enjoyed our trip but that evening decided to return to Lijiang in the morning. The festivities would be over, accommodation would be available and we liked the place, particularly the old town with its maze of paths, rivers and streams.

When we arrived there, we found a small hotel hidden behind a high wall. It was an old two-storey wooden creation built in the local Bai style, with all the rooms opening on to a courtyard filled with pots of scarlet geraniums and small trees. It was as if we were completely alone and was so peaceful we booked in for three nights. We spent most afternoons drinking green tea and catching up on diaries, and the days flew by.

On our return to Dali, Wu Ling went back to her school, Toshi booked into a guesthouse to consider his next destination, and I returned to the hospital to prepare for my move to the Medical College. My summer vacation had certainly been an unforgettable experience. We were three very different people with cultures that were poles apart yet we had gelled so well and enjoyed each other's company without ever having a problem. It felt good to be alive.

On last day of August, Bryan rang with some devastating news. Diana, Princess of Wales, had died in a car crash in Paris. The time in China was six hours ahead of GMT, and I guess we knew the dreadful news before many because much of the western world would be sleeping. Dozens of ordinary Chinese people came to me and offered condolences. Although Diana had visited Hong Kong she had never been to China, but so many people knew of her and said she was like a shining star, a beautiful princess, the stuff of fairy tales. At midday I met with Vicky, Ian, Bryan and Silvia in Dali and we grieved together. Days later I was more than a little surprised to get a brief glimpse of the funeral on Central China Television. The authorities must have thought it was an important event, as did so many other countries.

Vicky and Ian were staying in a Dali hotel for a couple of weeks, making arrangements for their journey to Australia. They were to visit families and friends before heading off to Japan to continue their teaching careers. On their day of departure, I went with them to the bus station, said my farewells and walked home with tears trickling down my cheeks. I had said goodbye to two really good friends. They were both genuine, sincere people and at that moment I felt quite alone and dejected. I would miss them dreadfully.

Chapter 20

It was the start of the new term and Sean, my VSO Programme Officer from Beijing, visited the college. This bi-annual visit was made to ensure all was going well in the placement and I was surviving. He immediately put me at ease with a gift of tasty cheese and a big hug. With the Foreign Affairs team, my new role was discussed at length and everyone was satisfied. The evening provided invaluable time to chat to Sean and catch up with all the news of my fellow volunteers in different parts of the country.

The Medical College was a huge concrete monstrosity on the edge of Xiaguan. It housed not only the two thousand medical and pharmaceutical students, but also all the staff and their families. The Work Unit, or Dan Wei, provided housing and political indoctrination, such as Marxism, Leninism and the Thoughts of Chairman Mao for the students. Permission was required for the Chinese residents to get married, have a baby, change apartments, or work abroad. Strict rules applied to those who merited either a one or two bed roomed dwelling. The permitted child was often squeezed in with its parents or even shared the same bed.

There were two entrances to the college, which were secured at all times by uniformed guards. These people checked credentials and decided who would, and who would not, enter this crowded group of shabby, grubby concrete blocks at any time. The whole place looked as if it had been thrown up with little thought; an institution, possibly designed by the most boring urban planner available. Near the entrance, a few trees had been planted and a concrete lily pool had been created. Occasionally fish would appear, only to be caught, cooked and eaten when they reached a reasonable size. A tall limestone pillar, ravaged by the elements of time stood at one end of the pool. This column provided hours of meditation for the Chinese as they gazed at imaginary forms and entered a world of fantasy. That's what I thought anyway.

A well-staffed medical clinic was on site. This treatment centre offered family planning for married couples, plus treatment and care for most minor ailments. The large teaching hospital attached to the college stood on the opposite side of the road, providing the care for more serious complaints.

There was a kitchen and a large self-service restaurant for the students. There were not nearly enough tables and chairs for the numbers of hungry undergraduates, which resulted in most of them squatting on the surrounding grassy areas with bowls and chopsticks in their hands. The canteen doubled up as a dance hall on Friday nights. The large area above the dining hall was used for films, plays and many different competitions. A football pitch, four basketball courts, a running track and a long jump facility were nearby.

The establishment was one of two medical institutions in the Province offering a five-year science based medical or pharmaceutical qualification. There was a lesser course, held in another building, for village or barefoot doctors, who were introduced by Chairman Mao during the Cultural Revolution, from 1960 to 1970. These people, often poorly educated farmers, had the responsibility of caring for those in isolated, rural communities.

The majority of students at the college were aged between eighteen and twenty-three years and came from mainly poor peasant families, with homes in any part of the huge Provincial area.

"I didn't choose to be a doctor," said Peter, one of the medical students. "It was decided for me after I took an exam when I was in middle school. But I love it here and will work hard. My family have very little but they are very proud of me and I won't let them down. Having very little money I will probably only be able to see my family during the summer or winter break. With care, I am able to eat every day. Not a lot, but enough."

Peter's situation appeared to be normal among the students I was lucky enough to get to know. They were so philosophical and I never met one who wasn't content with his or her situation.

Their accommodation, with the sexes firmly segregated, was in huge blocks, with four students sharing a room furnished with two sets of bunk beds. Most of their belongings including their duvets were kept neatly folded at the foot of their beds. Under the bunks, boxes crammed with stuff sat beside enamel bowls with bars of soap, toothbrushes and tin mugs. Small threadbare towels were pegged to mosquito nets and rows of washing hung from strings fixed to the walls. A small table cluttered with books and pens was often just about visible. The only lighting in each room was a naked forty-watt bulb. Toilet and shower facilities were at the end of the blocks. Conditions were cramped and inadequate, but nobody complained.

It was lights out at ten-thirty pm and after this time I saw many students poring over their books with torches or candles. At exactly six o'clock in the morning, the tannoy system came to life and we were woken by loud music, usually with the Carpenters singing 'We've Only Just Begun' or 'Ticket to Ride'. Sometimes we would hear Celine Dion with the theme tune from Titanic and the volume was always on maximum decibels. The students attended a half hour exercise routine before their first lecture, while I snuggled under my duvet for a much-appreciated thirty-minute snooze.

My new living quarters were on the third floor of a Russian-style block of apartments, with the stairwell open to the elements. The surrounding buildings totally shut out any view except the top of a single mountain. It had been well used by previous foreign teachers. The décor was rough and the flat was furnished with drab fittings, which matched the nicotine stained walls. It had two bedrooms, a living room, and a bathroom with some interesting plumbing just off the kitchen.

An immersion heater in a huge tank stood high above the bath. I needed to balance tiptoe on a chair to check that the element was submersed before switching the appliance on. Once the water was hot the episode would have to be repeated to switch the power off and turn on the tap. The fuse blew repeatedly. My neighbour, a chemistry teacher, would come to my rescue putting thicker and thicker fuse wire into the box in an effort to stop it blowing. The equipment and mechanism of the water heating system was a nightmare not helped by the on-site electrician, who would occasionally arrive and poke a screwdriver into the system without switching the power off. In spite of everything I felt fortunate to have any water heating at all, because most of my neighbours had only cold water supplied to their homes. In fact, the electricity supply throughout the whole flat was dicey and every time I plugged or unplugged an appliance, blue sparks would fly. On the plus side, the apartment was nearer the bus stop than my previous accommodation and within easy walking distance of many little eating-places, and I did have a carpet, of a sort, to cover the concrete floor.

A post room, which stood immediately inside the main entrance, became central to my life. It was always foremost in my thoughts and every day I used to check for something from home, no matter how small. My family and friends rarely let me down.

In the two and a half years that I lived on this campus I was never taken on a tour of the establishment. I was aware that pharmacy and medicine, both Traditional Chinese and Modern or Western, were taught, but I never really knew exactly what other courses were offered or what actually went on behind closed doors. How were students trained? Did they have cadavers to learn about the human body? I knew people were buried or cremated on the day of their demise, if possible, and few left their remains to medical science. It was important to be 'whole' when joining the ancestors after death and autopsies were rarely performed. I had certainly got a lot to learn. Sometimes it felt as if I was on a roller-coaster and I knew I'd have to 'hang in there' if I was going to succeed.

My interpreter friend Rumei did not live on site at that time, but she had previously introduced me to several of the English teachers at the Medical College so I was not alone, and I could still visit my friends at the Affiliated Hospital where I had spent my first few months. I was able to maintain my relationships with Chen Wen Jia's family and Yang Kaishun, the Trauma Surgeon. It was also fun to keep up my football skills and be given language lessons from the youngsters.

The Medical College was a well-established organisation governed by a president, five vice presidents and so on down the scale. Alongside this group was the communist element with another president, his five vice presidents and a host of others. I rarely needed to mingle with these individuals because I came under the direct control of David and Charles, the Chinese officers from the Foreign Affairs Department. David was Chinese, but told me he grew up in Burma and spoke

English as his second language. He was a wiry little man with beady eyes who never missed a trick. He was often a stranger to the truth when it came to 'losing face', a fear of losing dignity or reputation in front of others. This was usually at my expense and I grew to live with it. He knew exactly what he was doing. Had my second 'dragon' appeared to give me a tough time? If so, this one would be more difficult to keep at a distance because I had to be in contact with him most days.

Charles spoke perfect English and did possess some humane qualities. He was often crouched over his desk in the office he shared with David. He oozed smarminess and was the underdog, running and fetching at every command, always keeping his head down. But when the boss was away he came into his own and always offered help and support when I needed it. I understood his position and liked him.

Two senior medical personnel were also to be on hand to assist and advise me. Dr Shi Li Min, or Francis, as I knew him, was an English-speaking psychiatrist. He was a pleasant, quiet, family man with a gentle disposition. He had spent a year working in Scotland and had a good understanding of how we functioned in Britain and he supported me fully. Dr Ding Yao Ming, or Jimmy, was head of the Science and Research Department at the Medical College. He was good looking and charismatic, keen to succeed in whatever he undertook, and appreciated my input. The only other member of staff I saw frequently was Mr Ma, an ex-surgeon, who was in charge of the fax machine. He was middle aged and balding and always greeted me with a big smile.

"Peggy, you have fux," he would tell me.

"Mr Ma, it's not fux, it is fax," emphasising the 'a.' "Say fax, fax, fax."

He would give me a huge grin and say "fux, fux, fux." Nice one!

I was never able to get him to say otherwise and gave up with a smile. We both knew that every fax I received had been translated and scrutinised before it reached my hands.

With my new job came the allocation of a bike. I was more than a little nervous when I ventured out on to the road on my sit up and beg, gearless vehicle to join the hundreds of cyclists, all the time trying to remember to keep to the right-hand side of the road. I hoped the car drivers would show me a little respect and give me a miss when they coughed and spat out of their windows. I was fortunate, because they either aimed and missed or ignored me. The bike turned out to be a blessing and many happy days were spent exploring places, particularly the local temples, and having picnics with my student friends.

On a warm evening, I sat at a table outside my favourite hole-in-the-wall café, watching the world go by and the people around me. Live chickens, tied by their legs, were sitting quietly in wire cages. Fish swam happily in glass tanks secured to the walls, and dark green fat frogs jumped up and down in glass tanks at my feet. Poor things, they were unaware they would meet their end when selected by a customer at the restaurant, because the Chinese like to see, and often feel, their food very much alive before eating it. It was marginally better than having to look at the dog tied up at the door of the café around the corner. This would provide an expensive and supposedly tasty meal for someone with plenty of money to spare. At times, I wished I could have emulated the wonderful Bridget Bardot and rescued some of these poor creatures, but I knew I couldn't. Difficult for me to comprehend, but that's how things were and there wasn't much I could do about it. I also discovered that people stopped and gawped as I attempted to negotiate slippery noodles or the last grain of rice into my mouth with a pair of skinny chopsticks without spilling it down my front! Sometimes I felt a bit like a circus performer and quickly learned how to ignore the audience as some of them had never seen a foreigner, let alone watched her eat! The restaurant was full and the place was buzzing. The tables had chipped melamine tops and were adorned with jars of wrapped chopsticks, small pots of soy sauce and white toilet rolls sitting in yellow plastic containers. The cooking area, along with the chef, was blackened with smoke from the coal briquettes used to heat the woks. I settled for an enjoyable meal of finely shredded strips of pork, rice and a variety of vegetables, without the addition of heaps of monosodium glutamate (MSG). This substance resembled coarse salt and was used as a taste enhancer, or so they said! Maybe it was fine for the

Chinese, but it made me very thirsty and dehydrated and led to insomnia and nightmares for me.

On the busy road in front of me diesel smoke belched from the exhausts of buses and trucks. Small red taxis and scooters rushed in and out and overtook in blind spots. By some miracle they avoided collisions, not only with the bigger vehicles but also cyclists and pedestrians.

Tobacco grew in the area so I had a wide choice of brands of cigarettes that cost next to nothing and I settled for the Hong Mei brand to help retain my sanity. The local beer was cheap too, but it was all relative to the cost of living. Heaven knows what the brew contained because if I had enough of the stuff I would hardly sleep a wink at night. It was always worth it though, and sometimes it felt good to get legless.

As I sat, my thoughts drifted back to chain of events that led to the start of my amazing journey here to Xiaguan in China. I had become more or less accustomed to my new life and found it hard to believe I'd been away from Worcester for six months. Time had flown by.

Chapter 21

On Mondays, I was scheduled to go to a clinic in the city and spend time shadowing the nurses as they went about their daily work. This activity was difficult to arrange because I needed a translator at all times. In all, I was only able to spend a total of four mornings in this building, with Francis the psychiatrist as my interpreter.

The sixty-bed clinic was three stories high, had no lift and was exceedingly drab. Inside the walls were painted a dismal light green colour and the floor was the usual grey concrete which seemed to be permanently mopped by a little soul with a bucket of grubby water. The outpatient's department was on the ground floor, the surgical unit and operating theatres on the second and medical wards on the top. A ramp had been built to the rear of the building and this was used to transport sick people to wards and departments. Most of the patients had been transferred from county hospitals for treatment that couldn't be provided in these often small, ill-equipped units. On the whole, the patients were peasant farmers who had travelled great distances over unmade mountain roads, accompanied by a relative or friend. Sometimes they had been sick for many weeks and were weak and undernourished on arrival.

Dressed in a white coat and a hat that entirely covered my hair and most of my face, I entered this treatment centre, feeling a little like the fairy on the top of a Christmas tree. But the experience was good and went some way towards my discovery of what these nurses actually did. The senior nurse was Miss Yang who had attended my nursing course at the new Affiliated Hospital. She was one of the students who had participated well and she welcomed me with open arms.

"Prior to 1990, only selected women and girls became nurses," said my interpreter. "Some did a six-month training course and others learnt through experience. They were usually allocated a position in a unit or department in their hometown or village. Many are still in these same posts. Those who excelled received further education and promotion, and are now practising senior nurses, in charge of units or departments. These days all nurses attend nursing school where their training is science based.'

He went on to say, 'Like the doctors, most of these women didn't actually choose to be nurses, and their future was decided for them by their examination results at middle school.'

The working day consisted of three shifts, with full reports given at the end of each session. The turnover of patients was huge, offering little or no opportunity for the nursing staff to get to know people, let alone complete the paperwork. Relatives often slept alongside the patients, who were always fully clothed as they reclined in their beds. The family provided the bulk of the nursing care and brought in the food. Many times, I found it difficult to identify the patient from the relative, to the amusement of all concerned.

No general anaesthetics were given in this clinic. Spinal anaesthesia was administered for most operations and cholecystectomy, or removal of the gall bladder, was the most common procedure in the surgical unit. Keyhole surgery wasn't used and, in spite of large abdominal incisions, the patients were up and about on the day following surgery, and desperate to go home.

The medical block overflowed with sick people, many of them suffering from tuberculosis in one form or another. Unfortunately, due to nursing insurance problems, I was unable to use any of my nursing skills and much of my time was spent in the surgical unit helping the nurses as they frantically stripped and remade the beds for new admissions. Other nurses were office bound, doing paperwork. This was an enormous task because of the volume of patients admitted and discharged within a set period. On the surgical unit, I watched doctors undertake the changing of wound dressings and removing of sutures during their endless ward rounds. It was exactly as the nurses had told me during my nursing lectures. Soiled dressings were thrown on to the floor or left on the bed and not once did I see any hand washing.

The outpatients' department was the busiest unit. A constant stream of patients turned up, either with or without appointments. A separate area adjacent to this unit had a row of beds for patients to receive intravenous infusions of antibiotics.

They would stay for an hour or two, depending on how long the infusion took. This was a common treatment for an array of minor illnesses ranging from headaches and earaches to sore throats and chest infections. Doctors prescribed the treatments while nurses prepared and checked the medications. I watched these women administer the intravenous drips with complete confidence as they carried out the doctors' orders. The used syringes, needles, glass vials and infusion sets were thrown into a large bucket. I did ask what method was used for disposal of these sharps, but was not given any answer. I later discovered that they were dumped at the back of the hospital where local children found them and held grand water pistol fights. Also, I suspected the farmers collected their milk bottles from the same source!

The laundry was dealt with in the open air on the ground floor. Sheets and pillowcases fluttered in the breeze alongside washed latex gloves, always a disposable item in the UK. I knew that washed gloves were better than none, but I was reminded of the washing instructions of condoms that were given to all soldiers during the First World War, i.e. wash your condom before re-use! In a room at the rear of the clinic nurses counted and packed gauze dressings and instruments, placing them in special metal drums for sterilisation in the autoclaves. This was a familiar scene to me because I performed this same act in my early days of nursing many years ago, long before the introduction of pre-packed sterilised dressing packs.

A frosty-faced cashier had an office just inside the entrance of the clinic. I was told that those who weren't covered by insurance from their work units paid cash 'up front'. Nobody would want to tangle with the lady behind the glass partition because she looked so terrifying. For many it was simple. No money, no treatment, even if they were dying. Patients arrived at the clinic on foot, in taxis or buses, or on relatives' backs and they were discharged the same way. I watched as one man was carefully transferred from a door, which had been used as a stretcher, on to a bed. His friends had carried him for three kilometres after he had fallen on a building site and broken his leg.

Whatever task these nurses performed, they were skilful and caring. At the end of each shift we would get together as a group and compare notes. Miss Yang, the senior nurse proudly told me they practised Nightingale nursing methods and pointed to a certificate on the office wall, and I could see they did. This particular group of nurses certainly did work closely as a team. Bearing in mind the vast numbers of patients dealt with on any one day, each was treated with respect and individual needs were met as far as possible. Much time was spent with both patient and relative explaining the need for caring and how to perform this role. This clinic ran a good nursing programme, which encouraged teaching, personal development, self-evaluation and self-discipline. They followed the doctors' orders rigidly and perhaps didn't use as much discretion as I, a British nurse, might have done. In England, it was my habit to discuss a patient's treatment with the doctor, but this type of action was unheard of here in Xiaguan. The nurses knew their role was a combination of art and science and considered education an important part of their vocation.

During one morning session, I met a delightful old man, a Mr Li from the Bai ethnic minority group. He had been taught English by missionaries prior to the coming of Communism in 1949. Although he was extremely sick, Mr Li gave me a graphic picture of the changes that had taken place in Xiaguan and Dali during the last fifty years. His feeling was that life was much better now as most people had work of some kind and were able to feed their families and educate their children. He also told me some Missionaries from Scotland had opened a clinic in Dali years before Chairman Mao came to power. They called it the Gospel hospital and it stood in the grounds of the Number Two Hospital. It was much appreciated and well used by the local residents before it was closed down in 1951. He went on to say there are two churches in Dali as well. One is Anglican and the other is Catholic, and that they are still in use. This gentleman had certainly retained his linguistic skills and was very proud of his achievement. I thanked him and promised to seek out these places.

After Mr Li's discharge from hospital, I kept in touch and visited him in his home with one of my doctor friends. This adorable old man was dying, and I watched as he lay surrounded and cocooned by family and friends. Some remained at his bedside day and night. He was free from pain, taking odd doses of opioids to relieve his symptoms, almost allowing him to have a continual farewell party. When he died his family would seek the advice of a fortune-teller who would recommend a suitable burial plot on the mountainside. This was important for the well-being and fortune of his family. He would be laid out, dressed in a special burial outfit, placed in his red, ornately carved coffin, and carried manually up the mountain paths by strong pall-bearers. He would be accompanied by hundreds of mourners dressed in their best outfits and a noisy band of people playing drums, trumpets and horns.

He would be ready to meet his ancestors.

I did go and find the old Gospel Hospital and the Churches in Dali. The hospital was just inside the gates to the Number Two Hospital exactly as Mr Li had described. Parts of it had crumbled away, but the outline was easy to recognise and nobody disturbed me as I ambled around. Walking away I thought about the Missionaries who had worked long hours, caring for the sick and wounded with few facilities. They were indeed wonderful people and they had left their mark.

The Anglican Church was small and basic with a couple of wooden pews and a raised altar. I spoke to the caretaker who welcomed me and said a small congregation attended every Sunday. I would be welcome anytime, but I never took him up on his offer. The Catholic Church was a short distance away and I was greeted by the priest, who was an interesting French speaking Vietnamese man. As we walked through the doors, I saw the whole place was festooned with bright, sparkly decorations that stretched from a central point in the ceiling to numerous hooks on the four walls. Amidst the brightly coloured streamers he pointed out the Stations of the Cross and a number of other colourful religious paintings. A statue of the Virgin Mary with new baby Jesus in her arms was positioned near the Altar. There were about fifty chairs in neat rows for the congregation. The whole place felt peaceful and welcoming so I took up the offer made by the priest to attend mass on the following Sunday. Not being a catholic I didn't know what to expect and on my visit, I copied the dozens of parishioners and knelt on the rock hard slabbed floor. After fifteen minutes of listening to the chanting and in extreme discomfort I stood up, rubbed my knees and crept away. Once outside I decided it wasn't for me, but I did admire the devout congregation. Many of them were elderly and spoke a little English and they remembered the Missionaries with love and affection. A few weeks later I saw the priest again and over a cup of strong black coffee I apologised for tiptoeing out of his service. We parted as friends.

Chapter 22

Because the doctors and teachers were working during the day, my teaching sessions were to take place three evenings a week for seventeen weeks, with a break in the middle of the two terms each year. I was quite happy with this arrangement as it gave me ample time not only to prepare my sessions, but also to get out and about.

Some forty students were to attend the course. Some worked within the college as teachers, and others came from surrounding hospitals where they practised surgery or medicine, both Western and Chinese. They had learned English by rote during their schooldays and could read, write and understand the language. They were extremely reluctant to speak it and it was my job to help them overcome this problem. We were to discuss common diseases, their treatments and the nursing care needed. Lessons were to take place on the fourth floor of the Library building.

Just before seven o'clock on a Monday evening I set off for my first lesson. The students were relaxed and smiling and I didn't feel at all intimidated as I took my place at a small table in the front of the class. I had decided that the first session was going be a general introduction all round, as this would give me some idea of their spoken English ability. During this time, I hoped to discover what diseases and treatments they would like to discuss, because if they had the choice the classes might not be such a struggle for them. I made two basic rules for my classes. No spitting and no smoking. We would have a break of fifteen minutes half way through for a short rest.

I discovered the participants weren't all doctors and teachers. Two were tour operators, one was a shop manageress and another was a seismologist. It added another dimension to my role, and what did I know about earthquakes or even managing a shop? I decided to stick to the subjects I knew best: nursing and medical English. Each chosen topic had to be discussed with the Foreign Affairs team before I could proceed.

These enjoyable evenings flew by with me trying to ensure that everyone took part by introducing role-play. I had great fun with the blackboard and chalk too, as I was no artist! I spent hours learning phonetics, which helped me write the different sounds for them to pronounce and understand.

We spent many evenings laughing as well as learning, and most of my students made good progress. Getting a little tired of talking medicine one evening, I decided to tell them about my childhood. On the blackboard, I drew my family tree and a picture of the farmhouse, garden, car, animal sheds, the large fields and a tractor. I spoke about my family life, education and employment. I had left my school and family at sixteen and had set out to build a new life. They found that situation difficult to grasp and could not understand how I could have left my family unit when I was so young. They became really motivated and began to tell of their own early experiences. Their language skills were improving and they were slowly but surely losing their inhibitions. I suggested that, as a written exercise over the next few days, they could write about their own early days.

Later, as I quietly read their papers alone, I could have wept. Most of them and their families had made a great effort to just survive, especially the older ones who had grown up during the Cultural Revolution. Many had been cold and hungry, but their parents had struggled to ensure that they had an education. Now they had employment and the majority of them were helping to give their parents a better life.

Doctors frequently came to my flat on my free evenings to practice their English, or so they said. The majority needed to offload some of their concerns. From the gynaecologists, I learned about the high abortion rate, particularly among those couples who had tried for a second baby without permission, hoping for a boy. They told me that even in the remotest village there was a committee, usually the village elders, who knew everyone's business. Any woman who was pregnant for the second time would be reported to government officials and forced to have an abortion, often at an advanced stage. No anaesthetic was given and the baby would be killed with an injection before birth. It was unacceptable to be an unmarried mother and bring such shame on their families. Most of the students I spoke to didn't even think about sex on a night out with their partners, but these young people were reasonably well educated and were aware of the dangers. However there always seemed to be much activity in the bushes in the parks at night and it was possible that the 'back street abortionists' were kept busy. I was never given any detail of these dubious activities, nor was I ever told what happened to these girls if any complications arose as a result.

The doctors from the Skin Disease Clinics told me of the escalating numbers of sexually transmitted diseases, particularly gonorrhoea. These infections were easily treated, but at some cost, and most of the clients came from outlying villages and towns to retain their anonymity, just as they do all over the world.

Sometime during the course, we tackled blood borne diseases. My students told me that Hepatitis B was common in China, and indeed some students on the campus were receiving treatment. When we discussed the Human Immunodeficiency Virus, HIV, and The Acquired Immune Deficiency Syndrome, AIDS, which is said to develop when certain symptoms occur and leads to death, they wanted to know more of the clinical symptoms and transmission routes. They knew that the first case in China had been found in Shanghai in 1985 and they were aware that the disease was escalating in sub-Saharan Africa. They also knew that Europe, America and Thailand had many cases. This was 1997, and I had never seen any educational leaflets or posters regarding any sexually transmitted disease, let alone HIV, but perhaps I didn't know where to look.

I spoke about the problem in Britain and how it had been addressed by education which took place in schools, clinics and countless other establishments. The class was polite and every student smiled occasionally. But what did their smiles really signify? By now I had learnt that this politeness usually hid other emotions. These students were the same as the nurses, totally unable to express their true feelings. As I cleared up before leaving the classroom that evening I was puzzled and disturbed. It was obvious that there was a great need for education and awareness regarding this virus. I was aware of the escalating numbers of sexually transmitted diseases in the locality and the link with HIV, but how far could I take it upon myself to discuss this subject openly? I would have to talk to my boss.

"David. My students are keen to learn about HIV and AIDS. We were dealing with blood-borne diseases when this topic cropped up. They've asked me so many questions and I'd like to prepare a paper on this subject for them. How do you feel about it?" I asked.

He studied my face for a few moments before his mouth tightened and his eyes narrowed. His glasses fell off his nose in indignation and his face reddened as he stood up and shouted. "Don't be so utterly stupid, Peggy. We have no problem here. It's a Western disease because you people are so decadent. You must be aware of that. It's an evil and foreign thing you talk about and that's enough. Now go."

Reluctantly I walked out. I was in a predicament. The doctors wanted information and I couldn't give it. What sort of society was this? I found it hard to understand and felt like banging my head against the wall.

I was halfway down the corridor when David called me back. "You're right. They must know." he said. "You can prepare a paper but you must bring it to me to check before you use it. You will only talk about HIV and AIDS in a Western context, using your British facts and figures. Everyone knows you are from a promiscuous society, mainly because of the lack of close family ties that exist here in China. I will see you tomorrow. Good bye." and the door closed firmly behind me.

I was pleased to be given the go-ahead, and yes, I would use the British facts and figures provided in the information I had brought with me. Deep down, I wondered whether the Chinese people really were different from us, and somehow, I didn't think they were. We weren't too far from the concubine era when most men of some importance had mistresses, and habits don't die that quickly. I had already learned how simple and cheap it was to buy mind altering substances in the area, which gave rise to the escalating intravenous drug problem. Sometimes I spotted syringes and needles which had been thrown into gutters and in local parks small groups of young people sometimes appeared to be semi-comatose. My Chinese friends took me to areas where truck drivers spent the night after spending many hours behind the wheel. Some of these drivers brought girls from all parts of the Province and dropped them off in the city. Somehow, they would have to find a way home and had to use other trucks as transport. They would have sex on the way and take potluck on the destination.

On Sundays when I went to Jack's Café in Dali I would try and meet up with Jianbuo from the Number Two People's Hospital and glean information about prostitutes and their problems. Jack proved a very able interpreter. All this had to be done in secret; I didn't want to jeopardise this doctor's position. He certainly had the wellbeing of these prostitutes in his heart and he knew many of them by name. Massage parlours and hairdressers changed roles at night and prostitution was practised fairly discreetly, as I believe it was still illegal, officially. Dali and Xiaguan, along with most cities in China were changing. Young men were streaming in from the countryside to work on numerous construction sites and the women were there, ready to practice the world's oldest profession.

Books told me that Chairman Mao had almost eradicated prostitution and drug taking during his reign, but now young people were quickly learning about life outside China and attitudes towards sexual behaviour were changing. I also knew that HIV and AIDS was a delicate issue, especially with David, and felt I should proceed with caution. Visits made to the local red-light areas with Chinese friends and the information gathered there had to stay in my head, or be recorded in my little notebook. I always listened carefully to Francis, Jimmy and Jianbuo. The doctors who visited my flat kept me informed of the local situation regarding STDs. With poor hospital hygiene and the careless disposal of needles and syringes, the easy availability of drugs and prostitution, this area had all the ingredients for an HIV explosion. I really couldn't say how I felt publicly because I was never quite sure who was listening. My thoughts and possibly the reality of the local situation could only be whispered to the shadows.

I phoned Sean, my VSO programme officer in Beijing, to keep him aware of my progress. I told him about David's reluctance to allow me to discuss HIV, even though he had now granted permission for me to use Western facts and figures. This was a start and I would keep going.

On the brighter side, I was getting to know more of the medical students. Five of them regularly visited me in my flat for assistance with their English grammar and pronunciation, which was incredibly difficult for them at times.

"Of course, I'll help you, and in return you'd be doing me a favour by buying me a chicken and some vegetables from the market and cooking it in my kitchen. I've got plenty of rice and chillies." I smiled in anticipation and handed over some money. They were much better cooks than I would ever be in this country. And, sure enough once or twice a week they would prepare mouth-watering food and cook it in my wok, with smoke and flames sometimes licking the ceiling. For me, they prepared chicken without innards, heads or feet, and without added heaps of monosodium glutamate. At first, they thought it a little strange that I didn't eat the morsels that they loved, or appreciate the MSG, but quickly realised the food I liked, or disliked, was just another cultural difference and happily accepted it. I knew I had the better of the deals, but my ploy also ensured a few of them had a wholesome meal now and again.

They also loved my bath and occasionally I would let one of them wallow in the bubbles. It was a rare treat for them as they normally shared the communal showers in their flats. For me, it was a nightmare to ensure they didn't use all my luxury toiletries which I could only replace when I went to Kunming.

Chapter 23

Because I was providing British facts and figures of HIV and AIDS at the Medical College, I felt a great need to link up with Audrey, Kate and Peggy in Kunming - the individuals I had met before the start of my placement. I wanted to learn more about the HIV situation in Yunnan Province in the hope that I could eventually extend my teachings to local issues. I requested permission to be away from my place of employment for a week and set off on the night bus.

I found cheap accommodation in the dormitory of my favourite hotel, the Camellia, and was delighted to find that the whole place had been upgraded. The dormitory area was a vast room at the top of the building. Roughly thirty beds were squashed in, each with a tiny cupboard between. This was to be my home for the next seven days and with breakfast included it was good value. It was more or less in the centre of the city as well. My money didn't run to anything better at that time, and it was reasonably safe and somewhere to live. Travellers from different parts of the world arrived at any time of the day or night, so sleeping was not easy. Some knelt on the floor and chanted prayers at different times, while others slept, or rested on their beds and chatted. Nobody undressed at night, and keeping identity documents and valuables on your body was essential as you didn't know who your neighbour was. There was a quite a problem in the morning too, because there were only two shower units and two toilets available, so it doesn't take much imagination to visualise the morning rush, the urgency and the frantic hopping!

It was in this unit that I met an interesting American lady, Lilly, who was nearly eighty years old. Her husband had died a few months back and she hoped to achieve her life-long ambition of hiking around South-East Asia. Alone she had travelled extensively around China. On this day, dressed in sweater, jeans and hiking boots, she slung her rucksack on her back and headed off to the airport with a ticket to Bangkok on the first leg of her journey to Thailand, Laos, Vietnam and Cambodia. Unfortunately, I lost contact with her, but have often wondered if she ever completed her mission. What a fantastic lady!

My first morning was spent with Kate, who headed the Non-Governmental Organisation (NGO) Save the Children team in the city.

"I've been here a couple of years now," said Kate, "and our organisation focuses on care for both abandoned and orphaned children. We include water and sanitation projects, and currently HIV and AIDS awareness and education is high on the list. We do have a problem and a need to inform so many people. Ask me anything you want, our library is at your disposal," she said. "Have a bite to eat with me and I'll give you an update on the situation in Kunming and in the Province as a whole, as far as we know." I left her with a half a dozen books under my arm and a diary bulging with notes.

In the afternoon I went to Audrey, an American girl who was in charge of another NGO in Kunming: the Yunnan/Australian Red Cross Youth Peer Education for HIV and AIDS Prevention Project. Their aim was to prevent the spread of HIV and AIDS among young people by training facilitators of a similar age. "Hi, Peggy," she greeted me, "it's good to see you again. Come and meet Li Gouzhi. His nickname is Gorgeous because he is, don't you agree? Come and sit down and we'll have a good chat and later on I'm going to introduce you to a very interesting lady doctor called Dr Cheng HeHe."

Later we visited the Centre for AIDS, Care and Research department in the city and met Dr Cheng HeHe, the Vice Chief Director of the unit. This dedicated physician welcomed me and provided me with the Chinese picture of HIV and AIDS infections throughout the Province. "Anytime you're in Kunming, come and see me," she said. "I would like you to meet my husband and our son. He has just started University and hopes to graduate in medicine." With her words ringing in my ears, I returned to the hotel for a rest. I liked this lady and was fortunate enough to be able to work with her at a later date.

The following day Peggy, the American nurse who was with another NGO, Medicins Sans Frontières, invited me for coffee. We spent hours discussing the increasing problem of tuberculosis, all linked to the rising numbers of HIV infections.

"There's another group of people you should meet while you're here," she said. "It's the Salvation Army Team. It's within easy walking distance from here."

These NGO's were all looking into various aspects of HIV. I had no idea how each one functioned before I visited and I learned a tremendous amount in a short space of time. Each one invited me to keep in touch, promising help and advice should I ever be given permission to provide any type of awareness and education regarding the Xiaguan and Dali issue, as there was a problem on my doorstep, even though the Foreign Affairs department fervently denied it.

The week was not all work, thank goodness, and one morning in the hotel I bumped into a big, amiable English guy called Geoff. He had spent part of his army service in Worcestershire and over a coffee we reminisced about the English countryside we both knew so well. His home was now in Northern Thailand and he was the only foreigner living in that particular area. Periodically he needed to renew his visa and jumped at the opportunity to come to China. He loved Kunming. Life there was so different from his part of the world and renewing his papers was a wonderful opportunity for him to spend a few days in this lively city. We had VSO in common, as years ago he'd worked on an agricultural project with them in Africa, teaching more effective ways of farming. He felt that his previous farming experience qualified him to help some of the poor farmers in his village.

"It's so important to me," he explained, "to help these people retain and sustain their unique lifestyles, otherwise it will be lost forever. They are hill tribe folk, mainly from the Hmong ethnic minority group, or Miao as they are known here in China, and I'd love to introduce you to some of them. If you're thinking of coming to Thailand sometime why don't you come and visit me and get to know the locals?" He added that he sometimes taught the local children English and tried to help the people in as many different ways as he could. We sat engrossed in conversation for an hour or so before he left for his return flight to Chiang Mai in Thailand. I promised to spend Christmas and New Year with him in Thailand, with a visit to his home village as top priority.

Another day, I encountered a couple of English social workers, Sally and Mary, on holiday from the West of England. They were huddled over their guidebook in the reception area and didn't know which way to go. We struck up an immediate friendship and not only did I become their tour guide but I was able to explore the city in more detail in good company. Kunming was such a beautiful place. Dusty and dirty it may have been, with building construction almost everywhere, but around every corner we found a new jewel to be explored.

There were Buddhist temples with brightly coloured religious frescoes on the walls and dozens of scarlet lanterns lining the paths. Rows of little women in blue were burning incense and offering food to the gods as they chanted their prayers. A smiling gold-coloured Buddha statue appeared to be breathing the pleasing fragrance from the smouldering home-made joss sticks that surrounded him. We were enveloped with an enchanting calm as we knelt in front of him and paid our respects. A monk told us our fortunes for a small fee as we shook a pot containing inscribed bamboo spills until one fell out. That particular spill told all and we were assured we would all live long and happy lives. We hoped he was right!

The Minorities shop was packed with brightly coloured hand-made wooden toys and beautifully embroidered jackets, skirts, blouses and shirts of pure cottons and silks. One floor contained musical woodwind instruments created from bamboo, similar to the ones I had seen in Lijiang a few months earlier. We stood mesmerised as a shop assistant played tunes and, to his delight, we danced a few steps.

In the side streets, the cooks worked in open kitchens with smoke and flames rising from their woks. The low stools on the pavement provided us with good vantage points to absorb the ambience as we tucked into our noodle soup. Nearby, a group of young people were sitting on the pavement reading volumes bought from a nearby bookshop. This shop stocked some English books, classics mainly, with Charles Dickens and the Bronte's being the main authors. A dozen or so Agatha Christies books were on the shelf, but regrettably I had read them all. I searched but could find nothing that interested me. I was now heavily into modern Chinese history, post 1949. Books regarding that issue were simply not available to me in

English, possibly not in Chinese either. The three of us made our way back to the hotel for a rest.

The next day was spent making phone calls and linking up with the three VSO English teachers, Helen, Sam and John, who were well-established in Kunming. Helen, a retired head mistress, wore her long hair in an untidy bun. She had been at the teachers' college in the city for almost two years and loved it. Sam, a handsome young graduate from the UK had joined her in August and was still settling in. John, in his late twenties, had an outgoing personality and was full of fun. It was good to meet up with these people.

As always, all good times come to an end and before I knew it I was on the night bus, returning to Xiaguan with my HIV and AIDS information hidden in the bottom of my rucksack. I slept well and peacefully under my grubby duvet.

Back at the Medical College all was well. David had arranged for me to give presentations on British Nursing Models and Practice in two hospitals within the Prefecture. The first was at Mangshi, near the Myanmar border and the other one at Binchuan, north of Xiaguan. I was delighted for two reasons: one was the opportunity to spread the word of good British nursing and the other was to travel and see more of the area. Meanwhile I would continue the medical English lessons to the doctors when I was at the college, taking care to avoid the sensitive issue of HIV and AIDS.

Chapter 24

"Hello 007. How are you this morning?" I asked Mr Wang the college driver. He loved it and greeted me with his huge grin. In his Pidgin English he said, "Me, Doctor No," and laughed as he pointed to himself. This tall, handsome man was a true gentleman, and although he could speak little or no English and my Chinese was minimal, we communicated well with our eyes and sign language. He loved it when I called him James Bond or 007. His favourite film was Doctor No. He had seen all the James Bond films and was a real fan. Today he was driving us to Mangshi, previously called Yuxi on the border with Myanmar, a long and gruelling journey to the south of the prefecture, and at seven in the morning we were ready to go. Charles, from the Foreign Affairs Department, would accompany me, and Rumei would act as interpreter.

We left Xiaguan and followed a narrow made-up road out of the city and headed south passing a huge hydroelectric plant pouring poison into a frothy brown river. We were out of the city limits and the countryside was desolate and featureless. There were a few scattered villages but not much else. The good road surface didn't last long, and soon we were bouncing over familiar cobbled surfaces, which was no problem in a four-wheel drive. At one point, I looked down into the valley and saw hundreds and hundreds of men and women armed with pickaxes, spades and iron bars labouring away in small groups as they constructed a new road. In the distance, I could see just two Chinese equivalents of bulldozers. Labour was cheap, and there were so many people grateful for any kind of work.

Our first stop was at Yangbi, a small country town which Rumei knew well as she had taught there on completion of her teaching degree. We arrived to a great welcome by the teachers and their primary school students. We sat around the tiny village café and ate noodle soup and steamed bread as Rumei and her friends reminisced.

Back on the road, Rumei loved my keen interest in the scenery because every so often I would request a stop to take a closer look at objects and sights that caught my interest, and 007 happily obliged. Once, on the top of a steep ravine, I spotted a harness contraption attached to ropes that stretched to the opposite bank. It was a pulley affair, used by the local population to cross the ravine and the raging river below. I'd never seen anything like it, but Rumei assured me these devices were quite common in rural areas, and would be well used by the whole community.

Our next stop was in a tiny village with a row of huts selling hands of bananas and not much else. We strolled around and in no time collected dozens of them, but there was a limit as to how many we could actually eat. In the end, we had to refuse more gifts.

The next hamlet had a narrow, rickety old rope bridge with wooden slats which spanned a small river. Once more Rumei and I laughed and played like kids as we wobbled over the swaying structure, clinging to one another for support!

By evening we reached Mangshi, the capital city of the Dehong Prefecture very close to the Myanmar border. We booked into a hotel and were joined by the hospital president and head nurse. They took us for a wander around this small town that looked as if it had been caught in a time warp. The streets were wide and dusty, with groups of men waiting on the corners with their hand-pulled rickshaws. This sleepy place was home to countless mysterious Buddhist Temples and gold coloured Pagodas. Beautiful colourful peacocks strutted around as I was given a running commentary at the Buddhist Shubao Pagodas. They were named after Chen Shubao, 553-604, the last of the Chen Dynasty Emperors. Four pagodas stood under an enormous banyan tree, with roots and branches growing through the structures. Some thought the pagodas were cleverly built around the roots and branches while others thought the tree came later. Whatever and however it was created, it was an intriguing sight.

That evening I was the honoured guest at a banquet. This time it was fun as I knew what to expect. The food was delicious and I cheerfully made several toasts to our hosts. Local dancers and singers entertained us, and I felt quite mellow as I made my way to bed. Having drifted off to sleep, the sound of the phone disturbed me. In terrible English, a male voice asked if I would like a bed-mate. This was the first time I'd been included on this special guest-list and I shouted some obscenity, unplugged the phone, curled up under the none-too-clean duvet in my shabby room and went back to sleep.

The following day one hundred and twenty individuals attended my presentation. I found the hours spent in the clinic shadowing the nurses had helped me enormously and made my work much easier. Rumei and I could only use my homemade transparencies with Chinese translations on a projector, but with the frequent question and answer sessions we covered a great deal of ground. As always Rumei did a wonderful job, and through her unique ability the session flowed effortlessly. The health professionals were a lively group, appreciating the differences in our roles, and hoped I would be able to return to continue our discussions. I completed the presentation with slides of my local hospital and nurse friends in Worcester. The girls loved our hospital uniforms – blue and white trouser suits without any caps. All too soon my day in Mangshi was over, and after a hot spicy buffet in the hospital dining room we said farewell and were back on the road, heading back to Xiaguan.

The next teaching session in Binchuan town would take place the following week and I would to be accompanied by my two consultant doctors, Jimmy and Francis, as well as Charles from the Foreign Affairs Department. We set off with 007 at the wheel of the college transport once more for the hundred kilometres or so journey, this time heading north. The road was mostly cobbled, but again the scenery kept me mesmerised.

The leaders greeted us at the hospital. The head nurse was keen to know about British nursing, and in no time took me on a whistle-stop tour of the ageing establishment including the Mother and Baby Unit, where I was to learn more about the high Hepatitis B figures. All new-born babies, who were clear of the disease, were immunised shortly after birth, enabling them to live fit and healthy lives without the worry of that particular illness. My lectures on British Nursing were well received, and the head nurse vowed she would make changes in some of their nursing routines.

The Skin Disease Clinic in the centre of the town, provided me with what was possibly the most enlightening break of the whole trip. Previously this building had been a Leprosy centre and had been relocated from the mountains into the city. With education and modern treatment, people were no longer frightened of Leprosy and the clinic now treated more sexually transmitted diseases than anything else, especially gonorrhoea. The young, keen doctors and nurses were well motivated. They knew the local statistics regarding HIV and AIDS and wanted more information, but at that time I was powerless to do anything about it so left the subject to Francis and Jimmy. I listened to the translations carefully. One of these doctors said, "Yes, we have some men with HIV. They are mainly farmers who are into intravenous dope. Their lives are hard and thankless. Perhaps they see this as a way to escape the drudgery for a few hours. We don't know, but it's a major problem."

No one was prepared to tell me what happened to them or their families, and my questions went unanswered. I could almost understand the need to lose a few hours in a drug induced euphoria, tragic as it may well be, because life was particularly hard for many of these extremely poor peasants. On the positive side, this was a very busy clinic with each day bringing new patients. By now I knew that the term 'Skin Disease Clinic' was really a euphemism for Sexually Transmitted Diseases. I was not surprised and remembered how the same clinic was tucked away at the back of my own hospital in Worcester, as few folks wanted to be seen entering this particular department. I guess life is the same the world over.

The next day brought my presentation to one hundred or so individuals, followed by an evening meal with the head nurse and the hospital leaders. The enthusiasm of the head nurse and her teams, and their thirst for knowledge, impressed me greatly and I was more than happy to accept their invitation for a return visit in the not too distant future.

Chapter 25

Back in Xiaguan, I was busy making arrangements for my first the four-day VSO conference in Xi'an. I caught the night bus to Kunming and flew with Helen, Sam and John, the VSO English teachers working in Kunming. I was really looking forward to returning to Xi'an and seeing the people I had originally travelled out with from the UK, and finding out how they were getting on. I would also be able to talk to Sean about my changing role.

This well-organised convention offered many different teaching sessions interspersed with relaxation programmes. Visits could be made to a dentist, and a doctor would be available to discuss any health queries. The in-country VSO team also felt that more time was needed in Beijing for new recruits who arrived in February and August each year. They looked for volunteers amongst us to show the newcomers around. I jumped at the opportunity, joining a group of five or so to be 'buddies' for the next intake of volunteers in February 1998. I was surprised to learn that nearly one third of the group I had travelled out with in February had returned to United Kingdom before the end of their first term for various reasons. The remaining volunteers had been happy in their placements. We had all come to terms with the fragility of life in such a diverse country, and spent hours renewing acquaintance with colleagues. The conference was a good break and I certainly enjoyed it.

Back in my placement all was going well. My teaching sessions were pleasurable. We were all more relaxed in each other's company, which made life easier for me. We covered a wide range of topics and most of the doctors were improving their English language skills.

In December, Sean my programme officer, made his second visit to the college. I had received many requests from doctors on the campus for more information on HIV and AIDS and I was in a quandary. The Foreign Affairs Department had made it quite clear that I could continue using only Western facts and figures. Francis and Jimmy knew of the local problem and were in the process of opening a clinic in a red-light area of the city. They requested a nursing input from me. The clinic was to be a profit-making venture, the proceeds of which would be used for staff salaries and the upkeep of the building. Sean thought it a brilliant idea and produced what, to me, was the greatest gift I could have ever received, a book printed as a result of a joint symposium on HIV and AIDS held in Beijing in May 1997 by the Barry and Martin's Trust, an English charity, together with the Chinese Academy of Preventative Medicine. It was printed both in English and Chinese and the statistics revealed that Yunnan Province had one of the highest incidences of new infections in China.

My original role of improving inpatient care had changed beyond all recognition and I was grateful for the continuing help and support that would come from VSO, my medical consultants, and my friends in Kunming.

The doctors in my evening classes were desperate to know more about the signs, symptoms, and transmission routes of HIV. I could see them looking at each other and nodding as I told them the facts, and several were more than a little concerned. Interestingly, none of them had any questions for me, but they took copious notes and thanked me profusely for the information. I couldn't tell them what to do, but hoped to inspire them to at least consider HIV when making a diagnosis.

I still had no computer and rarely had access to one at the college. The only other one available was in Dali at Jack's café. It was a useless machine as it crashed frequently and wouldn't give me the information I wanted on HIV. I knew it wasn't all a problem with the machine and I came to the conclusion that China had the best 'fire wall' in the business, and possibly blocked everything concerning this topic. I knew if I was going to be able to provide any awareness and education on HIV I would need the co-operation of many individuals, ranging from the college Foreign Affairs Department and the local Health Bureau level to the relevant health authorities, politicians and organisations at provincial levels. I wondered if I would ever get around the never-ending red tape and bureaucracy, and felt as if I were being strangled, very slowly. I studied the book Sean had given to me concerning infection rates in China, and the true picture began to unfold. I lent the book to my boss in Foreign Affairs and his views changed completely. Once he could see that our area in particular had such a growing problem he became much more approachable. Francis and Jimmy were saddened to learn of the figures on their doorstep, but not too surprised. They were even more determined to get the clinic up and running.

The term was drawing to a close and I was going to have a few weeks in Thailand over Christmas and New Year, having taken up the invitation from Geoff, the Englishman I had met in Kunming a couple of months earlier. I sought and obtained permission from the Foreign Affairs Department to have a break and they dealt with my exit and re-entry visas.

Prior to my departure I was asked to investigate the possibility of an HIV and AIDS training facility in Chiang Mai University in Northern Thailand for some of the Dali Medical College professionals to attend.

Somehow, I had survived my first year in China, having never once seriously considered returning home. I'd experienced some tough times, but had come through. Before I took up this new challenge, I knew it was never going to be straightforward move in this culture, but never realised just how difficult things could be. There were so many rules and regulations, and this, compounded with such a formidable language, sometimes brought me almost to fever pitch. It was difficult to feel anything beyond being an alien, a foreigner trying to adjust to an extremely different way of life. Rumei and her family had helped enormously, as had some of the English teachers, in particular Melissa, Jane and Jerry. Two of them had visited the UK so knew a little of life outside China. I also became acquainted with some of the local Bai ethnic minority people, who had invited me into their homes. They taught me so much about their traditions, customs and culture which was vastly different to the ruling Han Chinese. At last I felt I was coming to terms with these diverse beliefs, how individuals lived, their behaviour, and why they did what they did. I felt I was beginning to understand things from their perspective and I hoped I would be able to continue.

Chapter 26

The day was gorgeous as I boarded the Thai aircraft in Kunming. The cheery cabin crew guided passengers to their seats and presented each lady with an orchid. This was to be my first visit to the 'land of smiles' and I was looking forward to it. In what seemed no time at all I was walking through the terminal at Chiang Mai Airport to be greeted by my new friend Geoff. He grabbed my bag, and as there were no regular taxis, we flagged down a Tuc-Tuc, a type of three-wheeled motorbike with two seats behind the driver. This scarlet, blue and yellow vehicle consisted of a windscreen and a roof and was adorned with multi-coloured stickers. After some haggling and friendly banter with the driver we were off and away.

"'We'll go to the guest house first and get rid of your bag. Then I'll show you around the city, it's manageable on foot. When it's dark we'll get another Tuc-Tuc and find a restaurant. You'll love Thai food, it's hot and spicy and I know just the place." Geoff explained.

The guesthouse was full of laughing holidaymakers of all ages and I felt totally stress-free. Geoff and I had booked a room. It was basic, but it was clean and had an en-suite. I knew that I would enjoy this short break and the company. Just hanging about with nothing important to do was a sheer delight.

There was a swimming pool, a couple of noisy bars and four resident house cats who chased big fat rats up the curtains and on to the roof-space.

The city had a magical setting. The Mae Ping River, with its carefully tended banks, flowed around the ancient city wall. Now and again we stopped to visit temples and saw gold-coloured Buddhas surrounded by ornate spiritual paintings and large sticks of incense. I watched as monks in saffron robes walked to prayer when the evening sun began to sink. In the centre of the city dozens of people were selling souvenirs, clothes and jewellery. According to Geoff the folks around us were a blend of Thai, Burmese, Chinese and Laotian cultures, and this was evident as street processions and dancing groups in fabulous costumes passed by. I loved the unconventional way of life and felt liberated; free for the first time in many months. In the steamy humidity, the mosquitoes feasted on me, so one of the first things I did was find a pharmacy and buy effective repellent, not only to stop the little devils nibbling at me, but to stop the itch and pain I was suffering. In this part of Thailand Dengue Fever was rife and I didn't want to fall victim to that horrendous haemorrhagic disease.

That evening was spent in a small café overlooking the river. As I enjoyed my first Thai meal, Geoff and I made plans for our visit to his home in the north of Thailand. During the next three days, we swam in the guesthouse pool, relaxed, soaked up the peaceful atmosphere and enjoyed the good company, food and drink. I told Geoff about the request for some HIV and AIDS education for the doctors from Dali Medical College and sought his advice. He agreed to help and since he could speak Thai he would be more than a useful companion. We visited the local clinics and pharmacies and all the responses led to a Dr Prakong Vithayasia at the Chiang Mai University Hospital. I decided to pay her a call when I returned from Geoff's home.

It took three days of travelling to reach the village of Ban Kuak where Geoff lived. The first leg of the journey lasted eight hours and I was squashed up and sweating in an overcrowded, battered old bus with no air-conditioning. I was quite fortunate I suppose, because I had a window seat, but the fact that there was no glass in the frame only added to my discomfort because of flies, mosquitoes and humidity. I was happy to arrive at our first destination, Tathon. The town was situated right on the Thai/Myanmar border and Geoff told me both countries made claims on it. Military personnel from both sides were never far away, but amazingly this presented no problem to the locals who crossed backwards and forwards at will to carry out their business. There was a clear unspoken message to us, as foreigners, we would be in serious trouble if we ventured over the border, whatever the reason! Myanmar was strictly off limits for political reasons. We had no visas anyway.

The town itself was a pretty little place lying on the banks of the Kok River. Geoff told me the girls around us were from the Hmong, Lisu, Akha and Karen hill tribes. They were wearing colourful traditional clothes and their headdresses were covered with small metal discs. He said that many, many years ago, these and more tribes migrated south from China. I was amazed to see that the women wore the same costumes as I had seen in Yunnan, particularly the Hmong people. A number of scantily clad children were shouting and playing in the mud on the riverbank. They were happy, very dirty but well fed.

We booked into a small guesthouse, where each room was fitted with a large fan, a mosquito-proof veranda and a curtained bathroom area in the middle of the lawn. After we'd unpacked we headed towards the bar where a noisy party was developing with a group of Americans. It was Christmas Eve; we joined the group and enjoyed every moment of it.

Christmas Day was spent nursing a bad hangover and trying to appreciate the beautiful scenery during the four-hour river journey to Chiang Rai. We were in a long-tail boat, so called because of the long rod at the back that holds the motor and propeller. These boats were long and narrow, about a metre and a half wide and incredibly noisy. Ours was jammed with ten passengers, and we sat opposite one another with knees bent, each position carefully considered, to keep the balance.

Halfway through the trip we pulled in at an elephant orphanage and after refreshments we helped to wash and feed these lovely animals. I got thoroughly drenched when a young elephant decided it was my turn to have a shower and sprayed river water over me. Then it was back on the boat to continue our voyage.

We docked at Chiang Rai to be greeted by a team of motor bikers, the local taxi service. Geoff took my backpack, and we set off as pillions on the back of two bikes. My so called twenty-minute journey to Ben's Guest House turned into a nightmare, as the driver didn't understand any English and dropped me off at a deserted restaurant. In the long grass, I discovered three English hikers sleeping. They were so high on drugs that they didn't even know what day it was. I made a hasty retreat.

I walked and walked in the stifling heat, begging for water from locals who couldn't understand a word I said. Eventually I did meet someone who knew where Ben's Guest House was and I gratefully accepted a lift on the crossbar of his bike to be greeted by a relieved Geoff. It wasn't till the next day that I realized the city was so huge. I might have felt uneasy if I'd had that knowledge before!

Most of the following day was spent in the back of a small truck, with stops that included lunch and sightseeing around the Golden Triangle, the notorious opium growing area where Thailand, Laos and Myanmar meet. We spent time visiting some of the ethnic minority groups, mainly Akha, who lived in the quiet little villages surrounding the area. Time, once more, for me to buy little souvenirs to add to my already overloaded collection! Late afternoon we stood on a hillside and admired the fabulous view of ancient temples and green valleys at the meeting of the mighty Mekong and Kuak Rivers.

A hot and dusty three-hour bus ride brought us to Chiang Khong, a small town on the banks of the deep, wide Mekong River. We booked a thatched chalet at a small hotel and sat by the river to enjoy a beer and peer at Laos on the opposite bank through binoculars. This was a controlled crossing area. Ferries, that resembled long, slim missiles, powered by screaming turbine engines, seemed to travel so fast, that the water they displaced almost defied gravity by pluming at the front of the boat as well as at the back.

We woke to a pall of mist, which hung low over the now silent river. Birds sang in the trees and bees hovered over the mass of flowers in the gardens. The mosquitoes had taken their toll of my arms and legs as always in the hot, steamy atmosphere, and after a quick visit to a pharmacy, I was ready to go, but not before enjoying a breakfast of banana pancakes and strong black coffee.

A two-hour journey in the back of a small truck brought us to the centre of Ban Kuak village, Geoff's home. We had reached our destination.

The village was small with a few bungalow type houses on each side of the wide dirt road. A narrow mud track led to a few older type wooden houses on stilts, the farthest away being Geoff's. Children were getting out of school, and a couple of young boys, of about eleven or twelve, sped noisily down the road on their mopeds as they made their way home. Smaller children clung to the backs of their pyjama-clad, scooter-riding mothers as they went to their homes. Others held hands as they walked in small, motley groups at the side of the road.

There was only one café, and the owner greeted us with a broad smile. So far everything had gone well and reaching the village had been an extraordinary experience. I felt easier when a number of villagers came to greet us and joined us for a coffee.

Tired and dishevelled, the pair of us slowly made our way up the track. I stared at the house standing some six or seven metres off the ground. There were six teak poles that supported the living accommodation, each one with a wide steel band fastened to it. A ladder was propped against the entrance door. This was the first time I'd ever seen, let alone visited, a house of this kind.

"It's designed this way to keep the bloody rats and snakes out," said Geoff. "The steel bands prevent any creatures from climbing up and we'll be quite safe once we're inside. I take the ladder down when I'm away."

I had to believe him, but was ill at ease as I wandered round the building. At one side was a small shed built with concrete blocks. I opened the door and found a twin-tub washer, a toilet, a large concrete tub full of clean water and a couple of old saucepans. A naked bulb provided the lighting. On a shelf, a plastic bag of washing powder stood together with a toothbrush and paste, a face cloth and a bar of soap. This had to be the bathroom, basic, but fairly user-friendly.

I climbed the narrow ladder and entered the house. The large room was divided into two parts, a living room-cum-kitchen and a bedroom. A huge mattress lay on the floor, surrounded by a mosquito net that hung from the ceiling.

"I got all this ready before I came to meet you, just in case any four-legged furry friends managed to get past the steel bands and use the bed while I was away!" remarked Geoff as we prepared a meal of sticky rice and vegetables. "I've invited a good friend from another village to join us for our meal. Her name is Nit and she's a teacher. She's had an interesting life and I think you'll like her."

In the distance, I could hear the purr of a scooter and soon it pulled up outside. "Hi" yelled a voice, "can I come up?"

Nit had arrived. She was stunning, with olive-coloured skin, dark eyes and a mass of intricately styled curly black hair. She was from the Hmong tribe and spoke perfect English. Her home was a short distance away within her small community. We whiled away the evening laughing, chatting, eating and drinking but all too soon, darkness fell and she had to go.

"See you in the morning. I'll take you to my school and you can meet the kids," she yelled as she mounted her scooter and shot off into the night.

"You have your shower first," said Geoff as I made my way down the steps and headed for the bathroom.

"Oh, and by the way, I forgot to mention that I have a couple of lodgers in the form of large iguanas who live behind the washer. Disturb them at your peril. They may well give a nasty nip if they charge up your leg".

No way did I wish to share my ablutions with iguanas, friendly or otherwise. I stared at the machine as I closed the door. There was no escape, I just had to get on with my wash so I undressed, dipped the saucepan into the cool water, took the soap and doused myself all over. With my task complete, I fled and returned to a welcome glass of beer.

While Geoff was keeping the iguanas company I made my way to bed. I crawled under the net, made myself comfortable and opened my book. Suddenly, the hairs on the back of my neck began to bristle as I discovered I wasn't alone. I peered over the pages and became aware of a presence and it wasn't tall, dark and handsome. All of a sudden, I was eyeball to eyeball with a big rat. I don't know which one of us was most startled, but this was certainly not my idea of a sleeping partner as I'd settled for Geoff. He may well have been big and hairy as well, but certainly preferable to this little beast. I jumped to my feet and yelled blue murder. All this revolting hairy thing did was look at me resentfully as if to say, "hey, you disturbed my sleep and now you're deafening me!" In due course, my saviour appeared like an apparition, dripping wet and starkers, dragging a towel in one hand and waving a stick in the other.

"Where the hell is it?" he shouted as he dived under the net and turned the rat into panic mode as it frantically looked for an escape. Eventually a truce was called when what had been a most indignant rat became a shivering wreck, having found respite under a chest of drawers. Obviously, it had somehow managed to gain entry and desperately wanted to make an exit the same way. Sleep was difficult to grasp that night, in spite of a large brandy and coke, for medicinal purposes, obviously. I thought each unfamiliar sound might be the rat trying to cosy up between us. I felt uneasy and tossed and turned all night wondering what on earth I was doing there.

Next day Nit arrived and we set off on her scooter to look at her Hmong village, which consisted of a group of wooden houses situated on a slope of hard packed soil. The ground floor of these dwellings was used for root and grain crops and general storage space. A wooden stairway led to the living accommodation above. A large open hut in the centre of the village built from bamboo logs was used for village meetings and big events such as marriages and funerals.

The buildings were eye-catching, but the people were even more so. They loved their bright, highly decorated clothes, and all the ladies wore colourfully embroidered blouses over black skirts. Silver ornaments adorned the headgear of both young and old. Nit told me they worshipped the Sky Spirit who, they believed, created both the world, and their way of life. Here in northern Thailand, as in China, these same people, sometimes called Miao were mainly farmers, and had a strict division of male-female labour. Their hard work, patience and independence had kept them relatively free from the stresses of modern life. I wondered for how long?

The five and six-year olds in the class were all Hmong children who spoke only their native tongue and Nit was teaching them Thai. She hoped one day they could go to the local school where Thai was naturally the language of instruction. We spent an hour with picture books and crayons, pencils and paper, with my wonderful drawings causing a major distraction!

Nit and some her friends joined us for drinks that evening. Another interesting day had come to an end.

Morning brought the inevitable headache, not helped by a promised early trip around the Laos boundary with the Border Patrol Police. They had offered to take me on a guided tour of this wild and dangerous area and I didn't want to miss out. At six thirty my transport arrived; it was a beautiful sunrise and my head quickly cleared as I boarded the jeep. An hour or so later my passport was checked and the time of my entering the region was clocked, just in case I never returned. I was grateful to be travelling with well-armed companions as by mid-morning we had entered real bandit country. It was the territory of the drug barons, and these men were heavily protected by their own kind. It was an enormous problem for the police. Murders occurred frequently, with no one ever being held responsible. Tourists were banned from the area, but of course the rule was frequently broken because of the availability of many types of drugs.

The countryside was magnificent with thick, green foliage everywhere. The police told me the dampness and humidity created an excellent living area for venomous snakes, scorpions and spiders, and it wasn't safe to take a stroll off the beaten track. Being told about the wildlife was more than enough for me; I had no wish to wander and sat tight! At times, we came across Buddhist Temples and stopped for the welcome tea always offered by the monks. Small hill tribe villages would seem to appear from nowhere and people would come out of their huts to greet us.

We lunched with a small community of Lisu people on the top of a mountain. A spring provided cool, clean water and we washed our faces and feet. The Lisu peoples' single storey bamboo houses were in a semi-circle at ground level. We visited the Spirit House in the centre of the village where a small shrine stood in a basic room for ancestral worshipping. The men were farmers, and apart from working on the land, they hunted with spears and arrows. The women wore colourful blouses and long skirts with skilfully embroidered turbans covering their heads. Skinny kids, all hoping for sweets, small coins or pens, surrounded us whenever we stopped. I was grateful to have been told about this and had brought of good supply of goodies. I'd enjoyed my day in the jungle enormously, and felt privileged to have been escorted around such a wild and woolly area with such interesting men. They'd been good company and full of information, and I was exhausted when I was returned to Geoff's house, safe and sound. He had been on a similar trip a short while ago, and he reminisced and listened to my tales as we ate our supper.

My short time with him seemed to pass all too quickly. I had hardly stood still and had enjoyed every minute of my stay, in spite of the rat episode. I was sad as we said our farewells at the bus station, and accepted his invitation to visit again. I boarded a new air-conditioned bus for my return trip to Chiang Mai with an assignment to locate the HIV and AIDS expert.

Chapter 27

From my previous enquiries I had learned of this lady's formidable reputation, especially in the professional field, and I felt more than a little anxious as I approached Chiang Mai University to hopefully meet Doctor Prakong Vithayasia. I was armed only with a small piece of paper bearing her name written in Thai by a kindly pharmacist. As an introduction it seemed inadequate, but it was all I had and I decided to go for it. At the entrance, I found a prayer room with a dozen or so pairs of shoes placed in a neat line outside the entrance. Gifts had been offered to a large garlanded Buddha who sat opposite the opening, and curls of smoke rose from the surrounding joss sticks. Inside people knelt, deep in prayer. Stillness and tranquillity prevailed and I felt incredibly humble as I passed on my way to the reception desk. I could only speak a couple of words of the language at that time, but a helpful receptionist gave me instructions to reach the doctor's office. The vast building resembled a labyrinth, and as I made my way through busy wards, along shiny clean corridors, went up in lifts, turned right, then left, I wondered if I'd be lost forever.

Finally, I reached her domain and knocked on her door. Speaking in perfect English she said, "I don't know who you are. As you haven't bothered to make an appointment, I'm too busy to see you," and slammed the door in my face. I was taken aback, but stood my ground and knocked again. "I'm busy. What do you want?" she asked.

I replied, "I work in a medical college in China, and I'm enquiring about training courses for Chinese medical personnel regarding HIV and AIDS. I wondered if you could help." She agreed to see me, and we spent the next three hours chatting together. This tiny, dynamic woman, with personality plus almost overwhelmed me. She was Head of the Clinical Immunology and Allergy section at the University School of Medicine. Her formal role involved the study of autoimmune diseases and research into Leprosy. She went on to tell me how she and her husband, Dr Vicharn Vithayasia, a paediatrician and Head of the Microbiology Department at the same establishment, were working together in the city's Marahaj Nakorn Hospital in the mid-1980s during the onset of the HIV and AIDS epidemic in the area. "We witnessed the horrors of the then unknown disease, comforting many of the frightened victims, who were wasting away from an alien illness that was producing such appalling conditions." Dr Prakong explained. "By 1991 the hospital's paediatric wards were overflowing with infants that nobody wanted to be involved with, even though it wasn't certain they would develop the disease. We tried to keep the families together with counselling, but often this was not possible because their sick mothers could no longer care for their babies. Something had to be done"

In 1992, with the help of a Swiss millionaire, the Support the Children Foundation was created, and four care homes were established to accommodate some children who had had HIV passed to them by their infected mothers. A number of local women were trained to administer medicines and tend their needs. This was so important for the survival of these little people who really only needed proper medication and lots of tender loving care, as all children do.

By 1997 a number of these children were ready for school and Dr Prakong told me about the problems encountered when she tried to enrol them in the local primary school. Other parents did not want their offspring to mix with these special youngsters, even though they looked and acted as normal. "It was as if they were fresh out of a Leper colony," she said, "it wasn't until I organised a visit to the school with parents attending that I won the day. It was quite simple really. I just asked the mums and dads if they were sure they didn't have HIV and, of course, none of them could answer the question truthfully. They agreed to let these special children be included in normal classroom groups."

A willing teacher was trained to deal with any injuries that involved blood. All this helped to ensure that these children would be able to enjoy a normal life. Even with all the education that was widely available so many people did not fully understand the transmission routes of HIV.

This husband and wife team worked tirelessly to inform the public of Chiang Mai about HIV and AIDS. They had produced two books, one an Atlas of HIV, with graphic photos of many of the infections that may be acquired. These colour pictures left nothing to the imagination and would turn most people's stomachs, but they were intended to help less experienced medical personnel with the diagnosis and various treatments. The other was a Comprehensive Manual on HIV Infection in Clinical Practice, also for health professionals.

Educational booklets in ordinary everyday language had been written for the general public, along with graphic, colourful posters. A hot line telephone number was made available for anyone to use if they had a worry, no matter how small. Monasteries were visited and monks were trained how to teach students prevention methods. These places often offered a refuge to people with AIDS, so care of the dying was included. High schools and brothels were targeted, with advice given on the use of condoms at all times, and a change in sexual activity was encouraged. Clean needles and syringes for intravenous drug abusers were made available.

By the end of that most enlightening day, Dr Prakong arranged for me to spend some time at one of her Chiang Mai houses to meet her husband and some of the resident youngsters. She also provided information on the training facilities for foreign doctors at the university, and promised to visit Dali Medical College in China, to give a presentation on how she and her staff had dealt with the HIV epidemic. It wasn't till then that I realised what a hard journey was ahead of us in Dali and Xiaguan. It would take time. My Chinese colleagues, Francis and Jimmy, had made a start with their outreach clinic, but it was still in its infancy.

Two days later she took me to a large detached house in an upmarket part of the city. The garden was a well-used play area with toys, swings and seesaws littering the ground. In the porch, a neat row of shoes was lined up, starting with tiny trainers and flip-flops through to adult size. I slipped off my sandals, placed them at the end of the row and entered the building. The squeals and giggles of happy children in the kitchen stopped all of a sudden and one by one the six emerged and stood in a little row. They put their hands together as if in prayer, bowed deeply and said, "Sawadee Ká", or "hello," and I responded accordingly. My first words in Thai had been mastered, and I felt honoured to have had such an audience. I was invited on a tour of their home, and although everything was shiny clean there was plenty of evidence that these kids had lots of fun. Some of them had been extremely ill with complications of the virus, but on this day, they were all well and laughing as they clambered over Dr Prakong to plant kisses and hugs on her face and neck. A happy hour was spent with me sitting on the floor taking part in their little games. I, too, was kissed and dribbled on by the younger ones as they crawled over me, managing to steal their way into my heart. As I took photos, the children cheerfully posed and smiled. I couldn't help but be afraid of what the future held for these innocent little victims. Would they all reach adulthood? Would the general public become more understanding with time and education?

As I made my way back to the guesthouse I felt a mixture of joy tinged with sadness. Joy that I had met such an incredible husband and wife team, who cared so much for these orphaned or abandoned children, and sadness that these same youngsters would never experience real family life, at least not yet.

Soon I was to return to Xiaguan, and as I tucked the comprehensive record of events into my bag, I looked forward to meeting up with my doctor consultants and David from the Foreign Affairs Department. I had bought two of the Atlases on HIV. They cost me more than two months' salaries, but I felt they would be worth it for my Chinese colleagues as the captions were in English as well as Thai. I had forged a link between Dali Medical College and the Chiang Mai School of Medicine and I hoped it would be taken to its full advantage.

Chapter 28

"Come," said Francis one morning. "Jimmy and I are glad you're back. We are going to our clinic. We want you to see what we have, and listen to any ideas you might have that will help us. It's only a short taxi ride from here and we won't be long."

I stood and looked at the small, concrete two-storey structure that was sited in a row of drab, grey buildings, next to shops and offices in the new economic zone of Xiaguan. It was a mere stone's throw from the large new hotels and guesthouses that had recently mushroomed. It was mid-morning and the place was your average busy area with people rushing around and living ordinary lives.

"This whole neighbourhood changes dramatically in the evenings. These dingy massage parlours and hairdressers are bathed in subdued lighting. The dress shops hang drapes to hide the stock, and curtained cubicles appear in the limited space inside. Loud music blares from unseen cassette players and young, scantily clad girls hang around the darkened doorways. The whole area is alive with groups of men who mill about in unlit areas or lurk in the shadows. You wouldn't think it was the same place." Francis said.

I walked into the clinic and could see that it offered treatments for a multitude of minor ailments. There were chairs and couches, equipment for intravenous infusions and racks of medicines, dressings and bandages. "As well as treating normal everyday complaints, we hope to give information on safe sexual practices and promote an awareness of HIV/AIDS, certainly to the prostitutes, but also to the general public." said Francis. "It's not a big place, but we do have rooms upstairs which are used for gynaecological examinations. Jimmy and I think this position is ideal for a clinic of this type."

It was clear that my doctor friends had selected a good location and staffed it with a team of professionals who were keen and friendly. The lead physician, a devout Christian lady, believed that AIDS was sent as a result of the wrath of God, but assurance was given that she was kind to the prostitutes, some of whom were as young as thirteen or fourteen, and encouraged her staff to behave likewise.

The clinic was basic. A grubby hand towel and bottle of disinfectant stood next to an enamel bowl filled with cold water. This provided staff with hand washing facilities as the single tap that supplied running water was above a squat toilet to the rear of this building. The first-floor room contained five beds, and a small cubicle which housed an ageing gynaecological examination couch. There wasn't a curtain or a screen in sight, so again, there was no privacy. Two almost empty storerooms completed that floor.

"People come with a variety of medical conditions from seven in the morning till midnight. Only a few prostitutes visit as they are too shy. The staff hasn't been trained in the art of counselling and that's something we must think about," said Francis.

As a psychiatrist, he knew the value of listening to patients and I thought that perhaps he should be the one to guide the clinic staff.

"Once one of these prostitutes has experienced a sympathetic ear and understanding, I think the news will spread by word of mouth, and the vital education will begin," I suggested. Our cultural differences were so great I could see I'd have my work cut out to persuade these people to accept my British way of giving all patients, regardless of colour, creed or employment, appropriate treatment of high quality. It would be difficult as well, because these people did not live the liberal lifestyle I'd witnessed in Thailand.

Over coffee, Jimmy and Francis told me about the more enlightened country girls who didn't want the normal life of drudgery. They would run away to city bright lights to look for work. "These girls are mostly very young and poorly educated. They aren't streetwise and don't know the pitfalls. Pimps are everywhere. They intercept these girls and force them to work in brothels. It's supposed to be illegal, but it's big business," said Jimmy.

"It's a major problem everywhere" I answered, "and there's no reason to think things should be any different here. People are the same the world over."

A week later I was in Dali with Jack and Jianbuo, my doctor friend from the Number Two Peoples' Hospital in Dali. We were enjoying a meal when I noticed two girls emerge from the shadows. Jianbuo approached them in the dimly lit street and invited them to join us. They looked anxiously around as they stepped into the pavement cafe. Even though they knew Jack, the café owner, by sight they were visibly trembling. These skinny girls, who were no more than sixteen or seventeen years old, sold their bodies for a mere pittance Jack told me, as he translated.

"I do have a boyfriend, but he's a drug addict and most of my money goes to him," said one, who I named JiJi. "I'm trying to save enough to open a hairdressing business in my home village when I return. My friend is trying to do similar. We're ashamed of what we do. Our parents think we work in a factory, and we'd rather die than tell them the truth."

What did they know about safe sex or HIV? Not much, I suspected.

"We ask for condoms at Dr Jianbuo's clinic and try to get the men to use them," she went on, "and we're always frightened when we are with our clients because sometimes they beat us when they see the condoms. Most of these men have very little money and they expect us to do whatever they want."

JiJi had been a prostitute for more than a year and I reckoned had been exposed to several sexually transmitted diseases on numerous occasions, but was too frightened to have a test for anything.

"If I had a blood test and the result was HIV positive, I would be reported and detained by the authorities who would notify my family. I couldn't bear that. I don't come from Dali, and have never applied for a permit to allow me to work outside my area. I would be in big trouble with the law."

My heart went out to this poor girl. She and her friend were fortunate in many ways because they knew Jianbuo. He would listen and help them in any way he could without being judgemental. I was developing a great admiration for this dedicated man and the essential work he was quietly getting on with.

Chapter 29

"Hi, is that you Peggy?" The caller was the other Peggy who worked with Medicines Sans Frontiers in Kunming. "I'm off to an HIV and AIDS conference in the capital in two weeks' time. There are some excellent speakers, including Dr Emile Fox, and I wonder if you'd like to join me? Let me know in a couple of days and I'll include you. The venue is near Tiantan, or the Temple of Heaven, and we'll be able to have a good look around."

I knew I would have to fund myself but jumped at the opportunity of attending such a seminar. Dr Emile Fox was the Director of the Beijing UNAIDS office and an expert with The World Health Organisation. I couldn't miss this occasion. I immediately set about seeking consent to attend, from both VSO and David in the Foreign Affairs Department at the College.

In due course Peggy and I arrived in ~~Xi'an~~ Beijing and booked into a small hotel. My friend allowed me to share her room, thus reducing my expenses considerably. The next two days were spent with me listening, learning and collecting as many booklets and leaflets, both in Chinese and English, as I could find. I worked hard and made copious notes. There were lighter times too, and the opportunity to meet and talk to Dr Emile Fox was one of the best things I could have done. This approachable man was full of valuable information regarding China and HIV. He was also interested in the new project at the Medical College regarding HIV and AIDS education and awareness, and offered to help in any way he could. We arranged to keep in touch by email, with me using a friend's computer.

Evenings were spent exploring Tiantan. This strikingly beautiful building was originally built in 1420 and had been re-vamped several times over the years. The round building stood on a square footing, based on ancient Chinese beliefs that the heavens were circular and the earth was square. It was here that Emperors of the Ming and Qing dynasties came to make offerings to the heavens and pray for good harvests. This sacred site, with its symbolic vibrant paintings, its geometry around the imperial number nine, and the acoustics that bounced off the marble balustrades left me dumbfounded. I found the ancient history intriguing, so different from anything I had seen or heard before.

I was well pleased with my two-day visit. New contacts had been made and I had been presented with another reliable picture of the huge HIV problem in China. I now had an even better understanding of the situation due mainly through ignorance, lack of material for training purposes and very little information for the general public, certainly in my area. How much would I be able to do in Xiaguan and Dali? As far as I was concerned the whole topic was still shrouded in red tape and bureaucracy. But the curtain was slowly lifting. The clinic in the red-light area had opened and I could see a glimmer of hope and light at the end of the tunnel.

Chapter 30

Towards the end of the month I would return to Beijing to do my 'buddy' bit of escorting some of the new intake of VSO volunteers around the city. My youngest son, Mike and his wife Lucy were coming out for a two-week holiday. I had told them of Doctor Yang Kaishun's need for the Campbell's Operative Orthopaedic Manuals and they were bringing the volumes as a surprise. I had decided that I would give Doctor Yang Kaishun a gift. He had re-set the fractured metatarsal in my foot and been so helpful during my depressions soon after I arrived in Xiaguan. I had never forgotten his kindness. Obviously, I couldn't do this for everyone, but I felt this particular man would appreciate my help. As I prepared for my trip I applied for, and got permission for one of my medical student friends, Tao Ran or Jasmine, to come with me to talk to the new volunteers as part of my 'buddy' role. She was thrilled at the prospect, having never been out of Yunnan Prefecture before. Her spoken English was good and she was great company.

Jasmine's parents were at Kunming Railway Station to see us off. She was so proud of her mother, a doctor working in a huge factory unit near Kunming. Her father, a slim, well-dressed man was an engineer in the same industrial plant. It was the first time I had met her family who, no doubt, were curious to see the woman who was taking their daughter away for a few days. I felt comfortable as I sat with this little family and was grateful to learn they had secured two hard sleeper bunks on the lower level for us. There were smiles all round as we walked through the station gates. We promised to visit them in their home with Mike and Lucy on our return from Beijing in a week's time.

We boarded the train, found our compartment and chained our bags to the metal luggage racks before making ourselves comfortable for the fifty-six-hour journey. The other four passengers in our compartment were looking at me with interest. They quickly accepted me after Jasmine's introduction and it wasn't long before the ice was broken and they started to practice their English.

The train charged through the countryside, which was sometimes quite empty and barren while at other times it was green and forested. Whenever we stopped at stations, a mob of vendors would rush to our open window to sell us rice or noodle snacks. At these times, we kept all our valuable possessions hidden away from the prying eyes. It would have been so easy for a hand to dive in and relieve us of our money, or anything else they fancied.

Each carriage had an attendant who tried to keep law and order in the confined space. Ours was a young woman who did an excellent job. She would come into our compartment every morning and evening and refill our mega flasks with boiling water. She would fling a wet mop around our feet at regular intervals and in the evening, she would tidy our bunks before putting our six pairs of shoes in a neat row. The small towels we used for freshening-up were shaken and spread carefully on a line to dry. Then, after a quick *'Wan'an'* or good night she was gone. At ten o'clock the lights were switched off. That was fine, but whenever we pulled into a station the full lights would snap on and the Chinese passengers, not renowned for their quiet and peaceful ways, would start shouting as they disembarked. Some ten minutes later the lights would be extinguished again and silence would reign as the train slid slowly, and almost silently, out of the station.

As always, the mornings came far too soon, and at six-thirty the lights would be snapped on. I would join a trickle of sleepy half-dressed folk and make my way along the corridor to the end of the carriage where a row of hand-washbasins stood. It was here that I performed my ablutions as usual with no privacy whatsoever. The toilet was of the usual squat variety, with a hole that drained straight on to the track that hurtled below. It was no problem for me. I'd experienced this before, but I was glad to find a door, even though it didn't close properly. Privacy, no matter how small, was always welcome.

Two and a half days after we left Kunming we pulled into Beijing Railway Station to the strains of Auld Lang Syne on the tannoy system. By now I had become used to the unexpected, and this was just another little episode to remember.

We were lodging at the same scruffy hotel I'd stayed in when I had originally arrived in China a year ago, and nothing had changed. The four other 'Buddies' were there and were delighted to meet Jasmine. The new volunteers weren't due to arrive till the following morning and the six of us had a great time renewing our friendships, catching up on the news, and working out some sort of a programme for the new guests. Three of the VSO Programme Officers were there too. It was good to see them again and discuss any problems that may have occurred in relation to work or health. I loved the fact there were no strict rules; it was a refreshing change from working at the college. We decided anyone of the new intake could join up with any Buddy group to visit whichever place of interest might appeal to them.

The next five days were both educational and entertaining. Jasmine talked non-stop and loved the attention she received. For me, well, I was just glad to have her with me. She was great company and did all the translating as my Mandarin was totally inadequate. On our first day, we headed for Tiananmen Square on the underground. It was cheap and far less nerve racking than any taxi ride! Jasmine wanted to pay her respects to Chairman Mao as well so we guided our small group towards the great mausoleum. We had to leave our valuables and cameras in locked cupboards near the entrance and were frisked before being allowed to join the seemingly never-ending queue. A great hush fell about us as we entered the dimly lit room. A glass-topped sarcophagus contained the embalmed body. Mao was dressed in a traditional suit buttoned to his neck and the body was draped in the national flag. I stared. There were so many questions. Was this the real thing? I knew he was dead, but this person didn't look as if he'd ever been alive. His face was puffy and the skin a bad colour. We couldn't linger, however, the guards made sure of that, and kept us on the move the whole time. Almost before we realised it, we were shuffling our way out into sunshine with the hundreds of other visitors.

Once outside, I looked around. This time I was seeing so much more. The vendors were still trying to sell their memorabilia, and the kite flyers were on top form, but there was something else; the whole area was monitored and I had been oblivious to all of this on my first visit. Police vans, bristling with cameras and aerials on their roofs, seemed to be everywhere. I suspected many police and guards were in plain clothes and some may even have been kite flyers. I watched as one van sped towards a small group some distance away. Without ceremony, this whole bunch of people were thrown into the vehicle and whisked away. I wondered what crime they had committed. I was to find out during my stay, that any kind of demonstration anywhere was forbidden; for those who tried, the punishment was unpleasant.

Jasmine proved to be an excellent translator and loved our jaunts. On numerous occasions when we got totally lost, she would keep her cool and guide us through. We spent hours in the Forbidden City, the Summer Palace and Tiantan Park, taking photos and videos. We jumped on and off the city buses at will and found intriguing places like the hutongs, or densely populated narrow alleyways surrounding Tiananmen Square.

Rows of three and four storey structures had the inevitable tangles of overhead power cables which hung dangerously close to our heads as we wandered along. We met whole families sitting in little groups, often with a baby and an elderly grandparent being cared for. We could almost feel the close community spirit as they beckoned to us to join them with cups of green tea. Clothes lines stretched high above us and washing fluttered in the breeze. Small pet dogs wandered about and quickly returned to their owners for reassurance when they spotted us. In these backstreets, we found good cheap restaurants and enjoyed Peking duck and the many other local foods which though mostly unrecognisable, were tasty.

The new volunteers were enchanted with Jasmine and listened to her stories in complete silence. She told them about her early days when she lived on a farm with her grandparents in Dali and about Chinese life in general. She went on to say that she hoped to be a doctor and follow her mother's footsteps.

On reflection, I wished I'd had the opportunity to share the company of such an interesting person when I'd first arrived in the country. The new volunteers appreciated the efforts we had made in escorting them around a few of the 'treasures' in Beijing and we felt the episode had been a complete success. I had certainly gained from the event.

An excited Jasmine woke next morning. Our 'buddy' episode had finished. We had got on extremely well as a group and had many laughs at the end of each day as we recalled getting hopelessly lost in our explorations of Beijing. We 'buddies' all parted as friends, but not before Judy, an English teacher in Guilin and I made arrangements to travel together during the summer holiday. Over breakfast we said our farewells to the new volunteers and, after wishing them well in their placements, we set off. Jasmine and I were off to the airport to meet my son Mike and his wife Lu.

The city traffic as always seemed chaotic, but our taxi made steady progress and it wasn't long before I was able to sit back and enjoy the journey that seemed so different from a year ago when I had first arrived in China. The trees had lost most of their decorative trimmings of pink plastic bags and rags, and many of the buildings alongside the road were completed and occupied.

The airport was buzzing. People were talking together and I couldn't escape from the excitement. I was on tenterhooks; the adrenaline was flowing and I could hardly wait to see my family again. Quite suddenly, Mike and Lu emerged through the gap, and it seemed almost as if we had never been apart.

The next few days were spent in a five-star hotel in the city centre, the luxury of which Jasmine had never experienced in her life. We shared a twin-bedded room and on several occasions, I left my student friend to spend hours up to her neck in bubbles in the bath, her first possibly since she was an infant. She thoroughly enjoyed the lavishness. When the four of us were visiting some of the Beijing sites, I was feeling almost like an experienced tour guide as a result of my 'buddy' experience, and was able to describe many of the places to

Mike and Lu. They loved it, and with Jasmine's help were able to see so much and have a good insight into Chinese history.

Because of the time factor, we decided to fly back to Kunming. This was to be Jasmine's first flight and we secured a window seat for her. I swear she never moved a single muscle for the whole four hours and this time it was her who was speechless. On landing we made our way to her parents' home and enjoyed their hospitality. Mike and Lu watched as a typical family meal of rice, numerous vegetables and meat and little dumplings was prepared and cooked, with smoke and flames licking round the wok. Like me they didn't recognise all the foods but we ate everything. There was the odd struggle with the chopsticks and hot, hot chilli, but we laughed till we cried. In the evening, sadly, we had to go and said goodbye to our hosts. We'd all had a good time and relived the experience we made our way to Kunming bus station to take the fifteen-hour sleeper bus ride to Xiaguan. This of course proved to be another interesting experience for my family.

The next ten days were some of the happiest for me in a long time. I introduced my son and his wife to my friends and we spent days walking in the mountains or sailing on the lake. Chen Wen Jia's family invited us for a meal and we met his granny, a lively little lady wearing her colourful Bai clothes. We had tea with Rumei's parents, and her father loved talking to Mike and Lu about England and our way of life.

Yang Kaishun, the doctor who had looked after my ankle when I first arrived, invited us to the Affiliated Hospital. It was now functioning but still largely devoid of patients. He took us on a tour around the paediatric and surgical wards including the Intensive Care Unit, which was not yet fully equipped. We walked down clean bright corridors with signs outside the rooms written in both in Chinese and English. Spittoons appeared at frequent intervals. These items were obviously an important part of the furnishings and I hoped people would use them if they felt the need for a good hawk, cough and spit. The doctor introduced us to his staff, many of whom I knew from my teaching days with the nurses.

That evening he prepared a meal for us. He didn't know the Orthopaedic Manuals he so badly wanted had arrived. Gifts were few and far between in this part of the world, and I wondered what his reaction would be. At the appropriate time, we persuaded him to close his eyes and hold out his hands. He had no idea what was going to happen as Mike and Lu gave him his wrapped presents. The poor man was almost overwhelmed when he took the paper off. The bit of colour he had drained from his face and for a moment I wondered if he was going to faint. He struggled for words and stuttered, "What are these?" He opened one of the books and sat with tears brimming.

"Thank you, Peggy; I can hardly believe this. These manuals are just what I need and I'm so happy. I'll study some of the procedures and you'll be more than welcome to come into my theatre to watch me operate when the place is up and running." he said, giving me a big smile.

The three of us were silent as we left his flat. The gratitude shown by Yang Kaishun had been so genuine. I felt the financial cost to me, and the struggle with the extra weight that Mike and Lu had endured on the journey, had been more than worthwhile. None of us were saints, but it felt good to have done something special for someone who had so little.

We spent hours in the local markets and tourist areas absorbing the local culture. Langer, one of Jack's friends, arranged a tour around Erhai Lake by minibus which made periodic stops in the little villages. This gave my family a good insight into rural Chinese life with its smells and sounds. This same man escorted us on a boat trip to Wase, a village on the far side of the lake. He advised us to look after our possessions as the hunting season for pick pockets was in full swing and we foreigners were prime targets. So, with plenty of tissues stuffed into our pockets we wandered around the market stalls and bought little souvenirs. Later, we sat in a small eating place and enjoyed noodle soup, with a family of piglets running around our feet. Tired but happy, we returned to my flat.

On another day, we took the minibus to Shaping, the small Bai village at the other end of the lake, well known for its local weekly market. We bought little souvenirs at some of the stalls before climbing the bank to get a bird's eye view of the whole bazaar. Once at the top we were confronted with a sea of huge red umbrellas covering piles and piles of red-hot scarlet chilli peppers. This clip was one of the many memorable shots recorded by Mike on his video camera and another one was a dentist pedalling a device that resembled a treadle sewing machine. This contraption supplied the power for a noisy dental drill, with a lady sitting on a white plastic chair. Later, this uncomplaining lady had a molar removed without a squeak or any local anaesthetic. There was no sign of water for mouth-rinsing or hand washing. When the dentist realised he was being filmed he left his patient and chased after Mike, but didn't catch him, thank goodness.

I knew a Bai minority lady called Jie Ling. she took me by the arm and said "Come with me". We went to her home to see her new grandson who was about eight weeks old. The baby was swaddled in quilted covers and cradled in a rigid bamboo carrier. When he was handed to me his little legs were bound together with bandages. Were they to keep them straight, I wondered? He was a happy little soul who smiled and gurgled at us. I later discovered that this was still normal procedure in Bai culture. There was nothing wrong with him and the bandages would be removed when he was a few months older. It ensured he would lie fairly still and not tumble from his carrier. Or so I was told.

Because I was still working in the evenings Mike and Lu accompanied me and took part in several of my teaching sessions. The doctors loved it and asked so many questions about family life and types of employment in England. Their English was improving and they were relaxed and chatty. We visited my college friends in their homes and sampled local foods and drinks and fell exhausted into our beds each night.

But eventually they had to go and I felt a big lump in my throat as I travelled with them to Kunming. I blinked back the tears as they checked in for their flight to Beijing to pick up their connection to Hong Kong. They were due for a well-earned seven-day rest prior to their return to the UK. As a parting gift, they presented me with a copy of Brassed Off, a British film of mining families who lived in a town in northern England starring Pete Postlethwaite. For some reason, the film made me homesick and would reduce me to tears every time I watched it. It became one of my most treasured possessions and, whenever I missed home, I would watch it with a large packet of tissues at the ready.

Chapter 31

Karen, a Canadian girl, had replaced Ian and Vicky at the nearby teacher training college. It was a pleasure for me to have someone to share the inevitable concerns that arise when living and working in a vastly different culture. She was a bundle of energy and laughed a lot. We gelled almost immediately, became good friends, and travelled locally as often as we could, sharing many happy times.

My medical English sessions of three evenings a week continued and it was rewarding to see the progress made by the group. An office had been allocated to me and I was beginning to feel like a semi-permanent member of staff as I moved some equipment from my apartment to this purpose-built site in a teaching block. The facilities were shared with the Public Health team who were led by Professor Yang Ting Shi. They were a friendly bunch of men and women who made excellent cups of green tea at frequent intervals and loved to chat when they had a couple of minutes to spare. I enjoyed their company and didn't mind when they wanted to practice their English, provided they helped me with my Mandarin.

"Peggy, you have fux. Come and get." A smile lit my face as I listened to Mr Ma shouting down the phone one morning. I still tried to get him to say fax, but he never could, and I didn't have the heart to tell him the meaning of his word in the western context and so he continued, and probably still does to this day.

The fax was about an HIV workshop, one of the first regional meetings on the subject, and it was influenced by the highly successful Symposium held in Beijing in May 1997. It was to take place in Kunming in ten days' time and would be partly funded by the London based charity, the Barry and Martin's Trust established in 1996 in memory of the late Barry Chan. Martin Gordon, OBE, was Chairman, and the aim of this organisation was to promote HIV and AIDS education, prevention, treatment and care, especially in China. I later learned Martin Gordon had been made aware of my presence by his niece, Nathalie who had a role within the VSO establishment in London. I was invited to take part and assist with the organisation of this event with Dr Cheng HeHe, the Vice Director of the Yunnan Centre for AIDS who I had met previously in Kunming. Two 'experts' from London would arrive to give presentations during the sessions.

I sat back and read then re-read the message and jumped up in excitement. Many of my local doctor friends including Jianbuo, my friend from the Number Two Hospital in Dali, were desperate to learn more about HIV and AIDS. Perhaps now my chance had come to spread some awareness of the virus that was so destructive in many, many ways. I was beginning to read between the lines, and could visualise the strands of controlling red tape and bureaucracy beginning to separate.

My visit to David, my boss in the Foreign Affairs Department, to get permission to leave the vicinity for a while was a pleasant experience for a change. Was this 'dragon' softening I asked myself?

"I'm very pleased for you," he said. "Francis will meet you in Kunming and act as your interpreter. If you need anything at all please ask him. Remember he'll be there to assist you."

He extended an invitation to the 'experts' from London, Dr Penny Neild and Senior Nurse Fiona Gracie, to visit the college for an informal meeting about HIV and AIDS. This would take place prior to the Kunming event. Dr Emile Fox at the UNAIDS office in Beijing was next to receive my news by email, sent on a friend's machine. I think he was almost as pleased as I was and immediately replied with the latest official facts and figures on new HIV infections in Yunnan Province. The numbers were frightening.

I was learning the secret of success, a system known as *'guanxi'*, loosely meaning communicating, or forming a relationship, with the right person or persons. I had made connections at local level within the college together with the relative medical personnel and important leaders. Now I was taking part in the first regional workshop of its kind at Provincial level and obviously had been accepted. My perseverance was paying off at last.

My head was reeling as realisation set in. There was a tremendous amount of reading and learning ahead of me. But I had tackled new topics before and succeeded. I was not too concerned. I knew help and support would be available from Audrey, Kate and Peggy, who worked for NGOs in Kunming, and one of my first moves was to reach Kate's library at the Save the Children Office to spend a few hours reading and learning. On arrival in Kunming I gratefully accepted Audrey's offer of bed and breakfast in her apartment for as long as I needed. It was a near perfect godsend.

The next week saw Francis and I huddled over the only Chinese/English medical dictionary we possessed in the college. Our greatest problems occurred when there was no direct translation for certain terms used in connection with the virus. In the end, we triumphed and produced a bi-lingual manuscript on caring for patients and families with HIV and AIDS. It was based on the holistic care method widely used in England. The photos of the Thai children would be included in my presentation. I couldn't think of a finer way to give an example of mother to baby transmission and the care these innocents needed. They looked so well and happy.

Chapter 32

In Kunming Dr Jiang Jiapeng, the director of the AIDS Centre welcomed me to his unit then left immediately for a meeting. He looked a trifle sour, and I got the feeling that he didn't care if he met me or not. He didn't speak English, but I didn't need words. The body language spoke volumes, and I was glad to see him leave the Centre for AIDS Prevention office in Kunming, leaving me and Dr Cheng HeHe, the lady doctor, to work in peace.

We studied the programme for the three-day workshop entitled HIV and AIDS, Clinical Recognition and Treatment. The speakers were to be Chinese doctors, apart from the two 'experts' from London and me. Dr Penny Neild was a practising Physician at Chelsea and Westminster Hospital, specialising in HIV. Fiona Gracie was Head Nurse of the Kobler Clinic, the HIV Outpatient Department at the same establishment, and I was to meet them at the airport in four days time.

There were so many questions I needed answers to. How much would the participants know and what would their expectations be? Their thinking was poles apart from mine. These doctors and nurses didn't ask questions as a rule, and although the invitations had been sent to the chosen health professionals, not a single person had replied with a request for any particular topic to be discussed. The first thing Dr Cheng HeHe and I did was prepare a questionnaire for all the participants. This would determine their level of understanding regarding the virus and would be completed both before the seminar and afterwards, telling us what they had learned. In this office, there was plenty of teaching and educational material, and the two doctors at the AIDS Centre had created several stations called 'Sentinel Sites' in Yunnan, mostly on or near the Myanmar border.

"It's where we take blood samples from known criminals, suspected drug addicts and prostitutes. That's how we get our figures on new infections," Dr Cheng HeHe said.

She gave no clue regarding care or treatment of people who were infected with HIV, but did tell me there was no access to anti-retroviral drugs at that time, possibly due to the cost. These drugs were becoming widely used in the West; they were not a cure, but delayed the effects of the virus and gave a reasonable quality of life to people like my friends in Worcester; an extension of life to get things in order and carry out whatever they had to do. But many people here in rural China weren't just poor, they were penniless. In reality, I guessed these people with HIV or AIDS were likely to be extremely sick and in need of tender loving care, regardless of their occupations. I would have to be patient and wait to discover their fate, if I ever did. In a Province, roughly the size of France, it was impossible for this organisation to reach every corner, and they hadn't yet touched the area where I lived. I suspected HIV was all around. The ingredients were there: intravenous drug use, little or no education on 'safe sex' methods, and sexually transmitted diseases, particularly gonorrhoea, were rife. A doctor told me that few, if any of the rural hospitals in the Dali Prefecture had equipment for blood testing, and in fact samples from Xiaguan were sent the 400 kilometres to Kunming for analysis. The general public had no idea of the risks they took with their lifestyles and I guessed that doctors like my friend Jianbuo in Dali were few and far between.

Friday was rapidly approaching. This was the day Penny and Fiona would arrive from London and butterflies had begun to creep into my stomach again. I had never met them before and wondered if my knowledge on the virus was sufficient. Over the last few days I had sought help and information from my friends and at times had been almost overwhelmed with documents and articles regarding HIV. Discussing prevention methods with Audrey and her team had been invaluable. I had begun to get a better understanding of the problem in China and how the Chinese were dealing with it, or not, as the case may be.

I took my place with dozens of Chinese at the arrivals gate holding my home-made placard above my head. I didn't want to miss these two people. In the distance, in a mirror reflection, I could see two foreigners approaching and I knew it had to be them. There were smiles all round as they emerged though the gap pushing their luggage trolley. Slim Penny with her auburn hair and brown eyes gave me a big hug. Behind her Fiona waited, her dark eyes laughing as I approached and held her tightly. It was a relaxed threesome which arrived at the AIDS Centre to be greeted by Dr Cheng HeHe and Dr Jiang Jiapeng.

I was pleasantly surprised with the clean, airy rooms we were given in the guest suite within the AIDS Centre complex. My experience of hotel accommodation in China up to that time hadn't been too impressive, but on this day, everything was fine. The group participants would arrive on Sunday and would be boarding in dormitories provided by the centre.

Penny and Fiona presented me with up-to-date books and articles on HIV and AIDS for my library. It was good to listen to these experts and update myself with current treatments widely used in the west.

I spoke of my class of doctors in Xiaguan and they wanted to know more. Their curiosity had been aroused when patients confronted them with illnesses they were unable to diagnose or cure and they were disturbed. I had become upset because I wasn't allowed to tell them all I knew. But David was my chief and I had to conform to his wishes or go home and I wasn't ready for that yet. My position was fragile, and I felt a lot better after offloading my concerns to people who really understood.

"There's a new clinic in the red-light area of Xiaguan." I told them. "It's the brainchild of the Science and Research Department at the Medical College and the two doctors who planned it desperately wanted to get it up and running. Its purpose will be two-fold: dealing with everyday health problems within the local community and providing information on safe sex and STDs to all, including the prostitutes. "Something like this is desperately needed, and I'm doing all I can to help them."

I told them about my trip to Thailand and my meeting with Dr Prakong. This lady had helped me so much and I would like our new clinic to run on similar lines to those I visited in Chiang Mai. But as they knew, it wasn't up to me and I'd have to fall in with the wishes of government officials, both at local and regional level. The meeting at the college the following day was going to be interesting. I wondered how many of my doctor friends would be able to attend and would they voice their concerns?

Saturday brought the 35-minute hop to Dali Airport with Yunnan Airlines. Excellent visibility allowed us to enjoy the views of the terraced mountains, which looked remarkably geometric from above. The sun glinted and sparkled on the windows of the village houses, giving a romantic feel to what must have been a difficult existence for the people who lived there. We touched down on the runway built on top of a mountain. Directly in front of us was the spectacular sight of Erhai Lake and the little villages that were built on the edge of the sparkling waters. A twenty-minute taxi ride took us to the Medical College.

After introducing my friends from London, I followed a smiling David as he happily escorted the attractive ladies to the pre-arranged meeting. Some fifty people were present, a mix of teaching staff and practising doctors from both the college and local hospitals. As we entered the room everything went quiet and all eyes focused on Penny and Fiona. With Rumei acting as an extremely able interpreter, they opened the session with a short talk on HIV and AIDS. I sat quietly and observed. The audience listened intently, but when the tutors asked if there were any questions there was an awkward silence. There was a great reluctance from the group to initiate any conversation at all, even those who had expressed a need to know more. What on earth was wrong? Then I remembered my nurse group a year ago and how many weeks it took me to bring them to life. Had the Marxist philosophy subdued this lot, too?

On direct questioning two of them said HIV wasn't a problem in the area as they had never met or treated anyone with the virus. On closer questioning, it became clear they didn't even know if there was any facility for HIV testing in the city. Eventually, a few began to open up and said they believed that the majority of patients admitted to the local hospitals had symptoms they couldn't identify and most were treated the Chinese way, based on observation and experiment, rather than theory. No one commented on the success rate. Someone said TB was rife and patients were usually admitted for three months to minimise infection and receive treatment. They were given a mixture of intravenous and oral medication. It was clear that HIV as a diagnosis was never consciously considered. At the end of the session I wondered if they would reassess their diagnostic techniques and consider HIV as a possibility with some of their patients.

Although the outcome of this brief meeting appeared negative, all wasn't lost. A year of working and getting to know these health professionals had taught me to expect little else from them. Penny and Fiona were amazed as they were used to western attitudes with plenty of questions and talk, both formally and informally. I knew they hadn't wasted their time and efforts; these doctors had listened and taken note. They would go away and discuss the subject in their own time.

That evening we were surrounded by a magical atmosphere. David, Francis and Jimmy took us to a riverside restaurant. The red wooden building had huge, colourful flower designs depicted on the panels. It stood in a garden full of shapes and shadows, illuminated by the reddish glow radiated from dozens of scarlet Chinese lanterns that hung from tall trees. We sat near the river for an aperitif and watched the fishing families as they tied up their boats in the fading light. I chatted to David, whilst Penny and Fiona discussed the HIV and AIDS issue with my medical colleagues who were keen to gather as much up-to-date information as possible. In the dining room, we sat at a table decorated with a red cloth and a bowl of red flowers. Above and all round were more Chinese lanterns. The lighting was poor and sometimes we couldn't see what we were eating. It was nowhere near the Ritz standard, but we all tucked into the hot, spicy food and washed it down with Dali beer.

Penny, Fiona and I sat up till the early hours and reflected on the day's events. They wished me well for my future at the college. Sadly, there was no time for sight-seeing in Dali. We had to return to Kunming on the early morning flight to meet the VSO programme officer, Jane, who was attending, and to prepare for the workshop at the AIDS Centre. Time was precious and we had so little.

Chapter 33

There was a hushed silence as the speakers entered the hall. The windows were wide open. The air was still and clammy and beads of sweat appeared on many faces in the audience. They listened intently and made copious notes as one by one the Chinese speakers hammered home their messages. They included the present known situation in Yunnan, China and the World, Chinese Policies and Rules regarding HIV and AIDS and the education of young people in the Province by the Yunnan/Australian Red Cross.

The workshop was new, radical in its approach to understanding and dealt with the problems of the virus. Each of the twenty-five participants was given the questionnaire Dr Cheng HeHe and I had previously prepared. They were asked to complete it before the workshop.

The Director of the AIDS Centre had the audience in the palm of his hand as he gave a report of the global situation. Solid facts and figures mixed with the individual emotions and feelings this subject always engendered. He dealt with the personal plight of those involved and the darker side of a world-wide social spectrum. He spoke with complete expert knowledge and ended his speech by saying,

"I realise some of you feel those with HIV should be segregated, imprisoned or hidden away from society or even shot," he said, "but this isn't the way forward." His face and body language fought the clamminess as he told the meeting HIV was first found in China in 1985.

"Today no one knows the number of infected people in our country. There are no real figures. Much of it isn't recognised or even recorded. But what we do know is that it is spreading rapidly and it is all around us. We cannot isolate these people and we must work towards an unbiased policy for all these unfortunates."

Dr Cheng HeHe dealt with the three transmission routes, all blood and blood products, unprotected sex and mother-to-baby. She spoke at length about strategies for prevention, both in the workplace and in normal living. She stressed the importance of confidential client counselling in a safe secluded area.

Penny and Fiona discussed the diagnosis and the many treatments available for the countless different symptoms. They explained how we had coped in Britain with the medical reality and the stigma of HIV and AIDS. They went on to say it had taken many years of open discussion to educate society into understanding the present position. Every patient was encouraged to talk openly about their problems in complete confidence, while the medical and nursing professions were tasked with prevention and treatment in a humane and professional way. While the situation in Britain was a long way from perfect, we had learned some valuable lessons, which could be shared world-wide.

My turn came and I built upon Penny and Fiona's presentations, focussing on caring for patients and families. I showed them photographs of myself hugging the children with HIV I had met in Thailand causing more than a few gasps to ripple around the room, as I wasn't wearing any protective clothing. This was again a wonderful opportunity to reiterate the transmission routes and emphasise the simple protection methods for health professionals.

At the end of the workshop I felt, and indeed we all felt, that our presentations had reached our target audience. The feedback from the questionnaires was invaluable and provided a much clearer picture into the future needs of the participants. We hoped those who had taken part were ready to go back to their areas of work and convince others that a positive programme was the best way to 'turn the corner' on HIV prevention and treatment. The workshop had been a success and grateful thanks were given to Barry and Martin's Trust for arranging and funding the event. Hopefully, the momentum would continue to grow.

Chapter 34

"I need a computer desperately, both for work and emails. It doesn't look as if the medical college are going to help, so I'm going to buy one. Will you come with me?" I asked Penny and Fiona. "I've never owned one and some advice wouldn't go amiss. I'll ask Francis to come as well. He'll surely know the best place to buy one. He knows Kunming well."

We headed for the area that sold domestic electronics. There seemed to be dozens of shops, all on the same street, all selling identical items. We searched and eventually found a Compaq laptop, the only computer with an international label. There were hundreds of cheap Chinese models, but I was wary because of possible problems when I returned to England. The laptop was to cost me more than a thousand pounds. Computers were expensive in those days. Both my bankcards were refused, but Penny came to my rescue with some short-term financial aid and I became the proud owner of a new toy and had to learn how to use it. Windows 97 had been installed, and with a little help from my friends at the college I knew I'd get by. Writing my lectures would be easier and emailing friends and family would add another dimension to my life.

We did a little sightseeing in the city before returning to the AIDS Centre for a farewell meal with Jiang Jiapeng, Cheng

HeHe and Francis. My friends from London had to catch the afternoon flight to Beijing to link up with the night flight to London. I was sad to see them go as I accompanied them to the airport. Fiona invited me to spend a day with her in the Kobler Clinic, the HIV outpatient department at Chelsea and Westminster Hospital, when I was next in London and Penny promised to keep in touch. These accomplished professionals had given me the confidence I needed. I now felt well equipped to support and assist with the new HIV and AIDS awareness programme that was shortly to start in Xiaguan and was overjoyed to receive a fax from the VSO office in Beijing telling me the Barry and Martin's Trust were happy to fund three more similar workshops in the Dali area.

Back at the college I sensed a great change in David's attitude. He knew there was a growing problem in the area and until now had probably thought it would go away. Full support was given in teaching the doctors in my evening classes, and he gave me permission to tell them as much as I could about HIV and AIDS. Arrangements had been made for me to hold teaching sessions and workshops on the virus at the Number One Peoples' Hospital in the city, as well as in the hospitals at Mangshi, Baoshan and Ruili, towns within the Prefecture, or county. I was more than satisfied and even more pleased when he said Rumei would accompany me to act as interpreter.

Chapter 35

I stood outside the College gates and searched for a western face. My VSO Programme Officer in Beijing had sent a fax announcing Simon Johnson, the Third Secretary from The British Embassy, with a special interest in HIV education, was visiting Dali. He would be staying for a few days and was keen to see me and discuss our college project. We had chatted on the phone with me giving instructions on how to reach the Medical College. I felt a ripple of excitement as I saw a solitary westerner in khaki shirt and shorts walking towards me. His face broke into a smile as he held out his hand.

"Hello, you must be Peggy. I'm Simon and it's really good to meet you."

"Welcome to our Medical College, Simon. I'll introduce you to David and Charles from the Foreign Affairs Department, and then we'll go to my flat where I'll give you an update of our project. Later on, my doctor friends, Francis and Jimmy have arranged to take us out for a meal".

Over several cups of coffee Simon explained his role. He had broadened his post to include drug co-operation and HIV and AIDS, including reporting on co-ordination and small project work. He was more than interested in our preliminary efforts at the college.

We spoke about the clinic in the red-light area. It had basic facilities and currently offered treatment for everyday health problems. He was delighted to learn I had been given the go-ahead to give talks on HIV and AIDS at three hospitals nearby, also that a study day on the same subject was planned to take place at our College the following week which medical and nursing staff would be attending.

During our lunch session, Francis and Jimmy explained in detail the aspirations they held for their clinic and invited Simon to have a look around. This would allow him to see the primitive conditions for himself. Both doctors expressed a need for some financial aid to get the clinic up and running. I suggested some involvement with Dr Cheng HeHe at the AIDS Centre in Kunming with regards to teaching the staff the art of counselling. David, my boss, who had joined us sat quietly and nodded in agreement. Simon listened intently and wished us luck before he bade us farewell and returned to Dali to continue his break from Beijing.

My role had changed beyond recognition. Providing education and awareness of HIV and AIDS was now my priority. As the first meeting was to take place in just over two weeks' time, my evening gatherings with the doctors were postponed. Francis and Jimmy were on hand, but it was really up to Rumei and me to prepare the material for our training sessions and ultimately gain David's approval. The college gave Rumei a break from her normal job of teaching English, and she needed it. A year ago, this girl had managed to learn about British nursing, and now she had to tackle the intricacies of a virus that was so unpredictable and invariably fatal. She studied articles in both Chinese and English and was intrigued. She had heard of HIV, but knew nothing of the real global facts and figures, or the damaging effect the disease could inflict on any one country, both economically and socially.

Gradually my friend took on board the seriousness of the message I needed to present. She understood how much I relied on her to get the points across to our audiences in the Chinese fashion, a way that she knew so well.

I studied the up-to-date information given to me by Penny and Fiona. Dr Emile Fox from UNAIDS in Beijing provided figures on the known number of infections, both globally and in China, while Dr Cheng HeHe in Kunming gave me the local figures. All this information I shared with Rumei, teaching her as we progressed through piles of paper. Hours were spent with the Chinese/English medical dictionary, compiling the necessary material for a series of bi-lingual lectures that would last a whole morning or afternoon.

"We have to make sure they all understand the wider issues associated with the virus and prepare them for the countless problems which may occur. We must also try to allay their fears and worries as we demonstrate the insidious nature of the disease, and at the end of the sessions we must measure the output, using the questionnaires and evaluations that were so useful at the Kunming workshop," I told her.

We emerged from our studies some two weeks later, well satisfied with our work and able to celebrate our achievement with a few friends at a local hostelry. Our first teaching session was to take place at the Number One Peoples' Hospital in Xiaguan in four days.

On the allotted day, a short taxi ride took us to the enormous, sad-looking building on the other side of town. The grounds were devoid of plants or trees and the inside wasn't much better. The walls were the usual depressing green and the concrete floors appeared to have been mopped so often they were shiny, particularly around the specially placed spittoons.

After being joined by the hospital leaders, Rumei and I went to the conference room at the rear of the hospital. On our way, we passed a ramp that zigzagged up the side of the hospital to the wards. There were four floors and no lifts. I stood and watched in amazement as a woman was carried up the steep slope piggyback fashion by a nurse. That was the way it was done here when there was no available trolley.

Preparations had been made for approximately two hundred participants, including three members from the new clinic in Xiaguan. Charles, from the College Foreign Affairs Department, was waiting for us. He had volunteered to be my assistant for the day and would not only be in charge of the questionnaires and overhead projector, but perhaps more importantly would be watching, listening, and learning.

The following four hours seemed to vanish. Rumei and I had done our homework and knew our subject well. We dealt initially with the virus, its history and the global problem. Some thirty minutes were taken up with some of the signs and symptoms. This was combined with a flurry of questions and statements. The transmission routes i.e., blood and blood products, unsafe sex, and mother-to-baby, were discussed at great length.

There was a deathly hush as I produced a condom, a Durex, complete with the good old British safety kite stamped on it.

"Hmmm," I thought, "they said the Titanic was safe, but hey-ho, this was not the time and place to worry about that, or the safety of the condom if it was misused."

I took the sheath out of the package and dangled it in front of the audience, explaining that if used correctly it was safe and could prevent most sexually transmitted diseases. Those closest to me looked as if butter wouldn't melt in their mouths, but many were embarrassed and lowered their heads. The women were more forthcoming and some even came up to look at the condom closely and feel it. At that time condoms were probably only available in certain clinics as I'd never seen them for sale. Why would anyone want one anyway? There wasn't supposed to be any sex before marriage, and I had been told married women were routinely fitted with a coil once they'd produced their child. And wasn't it only in the decadent West where sex took place outside marriage?

Two hours elapsed before we took a well-earned twenty-minute break. Rumei had coped magnificently and I congratulated her. With a huge smile of appreciation, she said, "This session is going so well. I can feel the audience relaxing. I don't think anyone has ever spoken to them like you and they love it."

With that information, my confidence soared as I walked on to the platform to share my personal nursing experiences with fellow nurses and doctors. I kept repeating the transmission routes and using the photos of the HIV positive Thai children, explaining there was no risk of infection from known patients, provided the correct procedures were carried out. As professionals, we could prevent accidental injuries with needles and sharp instruments simply by taking care during use, and disposing of them properly. In England, there had been accidental infections to both medical and nursing staff in the past, which led to ill health and sometimes death.

Time was spent on attitudes and feelings, both difficult issues to address within ourselves and in others because of cultural differences. We listened to some local values and beliefs and tried to dispel some of the local myths.

"People with HIV are ordinary people who will look to us for help. No amount of debate about whether the disease was due to negligence, ignorance or lifestyle will alter the situation. Most are innocent victims, they just didn't know." I reiterated strongly.

Rumei's continued ability to switch effortlessly between the two languages ensured the question and answer session that followed flowed smoothly.

At the end of the day I felt fortunate to be a British trained nurse who had taken full advantage of the further education available within our system. I had updated myself on a variety of topics, with blood borne diseases being high on the agenda. During a quiet five minutes, Rumei spoke to the staff from the new clinic and was impressed with their co-operation.

Tired but satisfied, we joined the hospital leaders for a banquet. There were all the usual local delicacies, which included crabs, prawns, black-skinned chicken and another big fish which, as usual, was placed in the centre of the table with its dead eyes staring at me.

The next day we studied the completed questionnaires and the results showed all the participants had increased their awareness of HIV and AIDS and, without exception, appreciated our talk. This was the stamp we needed and with David's approval, this paper would be the blue print for our future training sessions.

Chapter 36

Karen, the English teacher at the nearby teacher's college and I decided to spend the weekend in Weishan simply for pleasure. This small town lay some sixty kilometres south of Xiaguan and was home to many Yi and Hui ethnic minority people. It was well known for its Taoist Temples on the nearby Mount Weibao, and we looked forward to a different experience.

For our one night stay we booked into yet another small dingy hotel, the only one that we, as aliens, were permitted to use. After sampling the local noodle soup, we set off in a taxi to the foot of the mountain. Previously we had visited many temples together, and after exploring four or five in one day sometimes we were completely 'templed out'. But these sacred buildings were unlike any others we had seen, so the following six hours were riveting. Fourteen Taoist Temples lined the route to the summit and they were intriguing. The majority of these ancient buildings had beautiful spiritual murals depicting the many gods on walls, both inside and out. The eaves curled upwards towards heaven and were designs of pure simplicity. The vivid spectrum of colour was breath-taking, as were the carefully tended gardens. We met some wonderful people, some of whom were monks who had spent a lifetime there, and others who had chosen to spend time in a retreat for several weeks at a time or months if they wished. There was no time limit. We sampled different foods and had our fortunes told. We were given brushes and paints and asked to add to a mural of one of the many gods. We rested in tranquil and peaceful settings. Everyone was friendly and such was the atmosphere, I could understand why individuals would want to give everything up, live there, and free themselves from the rest of world.

Pain and discomfort woke us early. Too late, we discovered our mosquito nets were full of ragged holes and we were covered in bites. We'd missed a necessary check the night before because we were so weary and just fell into our beds. Such was the standard of the hotel, but in spite of the itching and pain we'd both enjoyed every minute of our short time away.

Chapter 37

For the next two weeks Rumei and I alternated our time between giving lectures and travelling to remote areas of the Prefecture. These talks had been arranged by the medical college and we were driven by our 007, Mr Wang, as normal. In one of the villages we stopped at I was introduced to some local delicacies including large white juicy maggots that squirmed in a bowl. They lived inside new bamboo shoots and were allegedly tender and tasty. I did manage to bolt down a couple of maggots, after they were deep fried and soaked in hot chilli sauce, but the memory of the creamy substance that filled my mouth when I chewed haunts me to this day. What seemed like hundreds of crickets were struggling in a plastic container next to them. When cooked they were tasteless and crunchy, and went down more easily with a large helping of chilli and rice. It was in this same village that I had to squat on a couple of planks of wood placed precariously over a raging river to answer a call of nature. A makeshift wooden hut had been built around the arrangement so at least for once, I had some privacy. When you have to go, you just have to take pot-luck!

At Mangshi I was greeted like an old friend. The audience was receptive to our talks on HIV and I felt pleased things had gone so well. Afterwards I was taken on a round of the wards and departments. They were airy, clean and tidy, possibly for my benefit. The patients, although startled to see a foreigner, smiled as I spoke to them in passing.

"No, we don't have any patients here with HIV or AIDS. They are in another unit." Rumei translated for the hospital leader, "and no, I'm afraid you won't be able to visit them, the nurses and doctors aren't ready." That was the end of the conversation.

Would they ever be ready for any stranger I wondered? I wasn't going to see anything or anybody. That was a certainty.

Baoshan was a small dusty town with a couple of shabby hotels. We strolled down dusty streets lined with beautiful, traditional wooden homes. Residents chatted in small groups at the roadside as they sold little savoury pasties and twists of rice bread. Grubby children ran around me, hanging on to my legs and begging for money, while their parents watched from a short distance.

The hospital was old, but had a pleasant atmosphere and here, my presentation was welcomed. The medical and nursing teams were approachable and open with their questions and I was elated with their reaction. Before we left, I was taken on a tour of a crowded outpatients department, but not before my camera had been confiscated!

"I've been told there's no one in this hospital with HIV either," Rumei said. By now, I knew I wasn't going to be told anything regarding HIV or AIDS patients.

There wasn't anything I could do or say other than, "Thank you for allowing me to talk to your staff. I really appreciate what you have done for me. Thank you again".

Once more I'd experienced the Chinese attitude that the virus was a western evil, spread by western devils or foreigners like me. Sometimes I thought their acceptance of this disease would almost be akin to losing face.

Ruili, our final port of call, had the feel of a real border-town about it with its mixture of Han Chinese and ethnic minority groups in colourful clothing, joined by traders from Myanmar. The hotels in this town were much more up-market, and the one we stayed in was clean, tidy and well equipped, a refreshing change from previous experiences.

A pleasant evening was spent in the market, ploughing our way through umpteen savoury noodle dishes and piles of delicious banana pancakes dripping with honey.

The squeals and screams of distressed animals woke me in the early hours of the morning. The damned hotel was within earshot of a slaughterhouse and the whole episode left me wincing and trying to hide under the covers. This wasn't how I wanted to start my day. I knew this unpleasant procedure had to happen, but I didn't really want to lie in my bed and listen. I resolved to get a room change as I showered and dressed, ready for an extremely early start to the day.

Rumei and I thoroughly enjoyed our presentations. Dr Cheng HeHe, from Kunming, had one of her Sentinel Sites, or special clinics here, and this group of health professionals were on the ball. They'd had many talks on the subject and were well aware of both HIV and AIDS and the associated problems. I was taken to a building, a secure government unit where people with HIV were held behind locked doors. I wasn't allowed inside, but at least these leaders admitted they had a problem and were dealing with it in their own way, whatever that was. Nobody would tell me what, if any, treatment or help was being given to these poor unfortunates.

Later that evening an incredibly thin trader from Myanmar approached me in the market area. He was selling a quantity of a dubious looking white powdery substance. I guessed any foreigner represented lucrative business for him, but not this one! When he realised I had no interest in his drug he reluctantly slipped away and melted into the crowd. In a way, I felt sad for him. He looked hungry and tired and was struggling to survive and in his eyes, he was supplying a need, as terrible as it was, and I doubt if he ever thought about or knew of the consequences.

These three hospital visits had taught me so much, particularly regarding the denial and social prejudice that existed against HIV infected persons. If my talks had made some difference, no matter how small, I would be thrilled.

Chapter 38

Back in Xiaguan the weather had changed and the rains had come with a vengeance. The air was still, and grey, heavy clouds hung low above me. It was sticky, humid and uncomfortable. What drains existed were overflowing. As I paddled along roads and lanes I wondered what unidentifiable trash was settling between my toes. Public lavatories were few and far between, and in rural areas many people answered the call of nature wherever they were. But I was fit and well, having never had a health problem in my time spent in China. Maybe my days of communal living in nurses' homes and subsequent rundown flats I'd shared with friends had stood me in good stead. I would never know.

I was deep in preparations for another three-day seminar on HIV and AIDS to be held at the Medical College in June. It would be funded by the Barry and Martin's Trust and speakers would include Audrey and Li Guozhi from the NGO Yunnan/Australian Red Cross in Kunming, and experts drawn from our own college. Ninety local health professionals had been invited to attend and I was delighted to find my friend Jianbuo from Dali Number One Peoples' Hospital on the list.

Because I was on home territory and presenting only one paper, I was able to watch, listen and learn. I had updated my papers with new information received from both Dr Cheng HeHe and Dr Emile Fox and felt confident. After the participants had completed the usual questionnaire regarding their existing knowledge, the day began with a question and answer session. Some said they felt HIV and AIDS was purely a social problem, and few would be prepared to help victims due to ignorance and fear. Others thought infected people should be imprisoned, or detained in a secure government building somewhere, to be ignored and never seen again.

Audrey and Li Guozhi spoke for two hours, and following a short break for lunch our own specialists came into action. At the end of the day the questionnaire was completed for a second time and we could see how attitudes had changed.

On the third and final day, more than three hundred students squeezed themselves into the lecture room for a lively morning session with Audrey and Li Guozhi. These youngsters were different from the qualified personnel and had enquiring minds. There were many questions and there was never a dull moment. Sadly, another session with students was never permitted during my whole stay, but those who managed to attend this talk were more than satisfied.

For me, the whole experience was humbling. I was beginning to understand more of the workings of these Chinese minds and knew it required a lot of guts for any one of these shy, introvert individuals to stand up and make a contribution, no matter how insignificant it might have been. I felt some were beginning to accept there was a problem.

Chapter 39

The summer vacation had arrived and I was going to spend a few days with Judy, a VSO teacher whose placement was in the city of Guilin in Guanxi Province. I took my usual sleeper bus journey to Kunming and made my way to the airport for the eighty-five-minute flight. The rain was hammering down as the plane landed and I got soaked to the skin as I splashed through outsized puddles that sat on the tarmac leading to the arrivals terminal. With water dripping down my neck, I fumbled for my documents to go through security control. This was not the way I planned to arrive, but what the hell. I was looking forward to the western company and seeing something more of this captivating country.

"I'm sorry I'm a bit late," a flustered Judy panted as she ran towards me. "My teaching session overran, and I didn't think I'd ever get here. Let's get a taxi and get you back to my place as soon as we can so you can dry off."

She lived within the grounds of a teachers' college where she was employed. Her job came with a flat that was similar to mine: drab, with nicotine stained walls and minimal comforts, so I felt at ease. It was almost home from home.

"I'm really glad you could come because have I got some places to show you. The limestone karst peaks are amazing.

Some go straight up and are very tall whilst others are in clusters. They come in all shapes and sizes. The Chinese love them and spend hours just staring and going off into their own little worlds, as I'm sure you know they do. There are underground streams and deep potholes under these structures too, but the mere thought of actually going down a big, black watery hole does nothing for me. But some people like this type of activity and these places are very popular. I can't wait for it to stop raining because you and I are going on a boat trip so you can see it all for yourself."

Sure enough, the rain cleared, and as we walked towards the river we passed a number of smart new hotels with gardens that were neat and well laid out, almost manicured. This city was obviously popular with tourists and all very different from Xiaguan. The humidity made me feel hot and sticky and I was glad to pause at a riverside café for a welcome beer.

We booked a sight-seeing tour on a ferryboat and boarded with about two hundred Chinese, probably mostly tourists. We cruised up and down the wide River Li for an hour or so and I studied the strange limestone formations which rose high and straight out of the water. They were covered in greenery, with the tops of the tall ones shrouded in a fine mist. We laughed and chatted to our travelling companions, trying to decide what these strange shapes resembled

"It's a good job you can't smell anything," whispered Judy. "The smell of some of these unwashed bodies is sometimes a bit overpowering, but I guess we'll survive.

Fortunately, the stiff breeze keeps it moving so it's just bearable."

Huge caverns appeared at intervals along the water line, with interiors that looked black and fear-provoking. I guessed the more intrepid amongst us would feel the need to go inside, but I agreed with Judy, it was all a bit scary and definitely not for us. Passing our boat were local men and women carrying out their daily work. The engines of their long narrow canopy boats chugged away furiously, leaving a frothy wave in their wake. It was a warm afternoon as the humidity had vanished once we started cruising and was certainly an idyllic spot to while away a few hours.

Next day we took the bus for the one-and-a-half-hour journey to Yangshuo. This small town was a favourite with backpackers and was buzzing with activity. It was similar to Dali in many ways with a laid-back atmosphere and smiling faces. The English-speaking café owners played Bob Marley songs over and over again, hoping to tempt us inside to try their western dishes and possibly buy some of the drugs most of them kept under their counters. We hired bikes and pedalled leisurely through narrow lanes and shallow streams, stopping now and again for cups of green tea offered by curious villagers. The afternoon was spent soaking up the sunshine in Yangzhou and drinking good cold beers, appreciating both the company of each other and the numerous western hikers we met. This was a welcome break from the normal daily frustrations we both suffered during our working time and had learnt to tolerate.

That evening we considered our next move. We had four weeks to spare and had saved quite a lot of money from our meagre earnings. The flight to Kunming was relatively cheap, and was preferable to the long tedious train journey. Our plan was to spend a few days in Kunming, chill out in Xiaguan and Dali, then travel north to Zhongdian before heading down to Xishuangbanna in the south of Yunnan Province. The remainder of our holiday would be spent in northern Thailand. Most journeys in China could be made by bus. It would be time consuming, but the invaluable experience would make the most of these in-country expeditions. We decided to make an early start in the morning.

There wasn't a cloud in the sky as we took off from Guilin on China Southern Airlines. The cabin crew, all female, looked attractive in their neat uniforms, but not one of them smiled. In fact, they all looked totally fed-up with their lot, going about their work of ordering passengers to their allocated seats like robots receiving orders from above. A hand thrust a can of jellied fruit juice into my lap without a word. I drank the odd lumpy sweet liquid and returned the can to the hand still waiting at my side, and then we landed.

Kunming was hot and dusty. Road works were continuing as was the construction of numerous high-rise apartments, hotels and shopping malls, and the taxi ride to the Camellia Hotel took twice as long as usual because of diversions. After checking into a two-bedded room we made for a nearby bar to quench our thirsts and just sit and rest. I loved the upmarket buzz of this colourful city and felt almost at home. I was more than happy to spend a couple of days there.

Two days later the sleeper bus journey to Xiaguan took just over twenty hours. Road works for the new highway were in full swing, giving our two drivers continual problems. We had to spend most of the time cooped up in our lower double bunk bed as the bus lurched round potholes and climbed steep slopes. We weren't alone because the thirty or so Chinese passengers were suffering in the same way, but nobody complained, well, except Judy.

"Bloody hell Pegs, I can stand the coughing and the gobbing out of the windows, and the rancid body odour, but these stinking feet behind us are something else. You are so lucky to be totally oblivious of it all, but on the other hand you don't know what you're missing. How much longer will we have to stay in this bus?" she asked with a wry smile as she settled herself beside me. I couldn't give her the answer!

Regular comfort stops were made at designated stations where white tiled pavilions had been erected. On payment for entry you were issued with one piece of toilet paper and directed to a row of cubicles with waist high wooden screens on either side. This provided a little unexpected privacy for a change. A tiled channel ran through them, and should you be squatting when the grand flush occurred, it was either your good luck, or bad, depending on which way you thought about

247

it, and once more I was glad to have no sense of smell. There were wash-hand basins with bars of hard soap and paper towels as you left the building. Whatever, it was certainly a great improvement on squatting down behind the bus. It was good to have a little walkabout to stretch our legs as well. We bought snacks from vendors parked next to the coaches and kept a good eye on our transport. With twenty or so parked buses, all blue and looking identical, we didn't particularly want to end up in the wrong one.

In Xiaguan we visited many of my friends, spending carefree days looking around Dali and enjoying Jack and Stella's food in their restaurant. We spoke to the local Bai ethnic minority women as they sold their wares, usually clothes and silver charms. They whispered about their stash of mind-altering drugs, openly offering cannabis seeds. Yi ethnic girls were selling similar goods, but were too shy to talk. They all wore their colourful outfits and looked striking. During a visit to Shaping market we rummaged about on the overcrowded stalls and bought too many trinkets. When my Bai friend, Jie Ling, offered us lunch at her house we jumped at it. Judy had heard about the ethnic minority groups in Yunnan, but had never seen them before, and was overjoyed to spend a short time with them and learn a little of their culture.

With so many places to visit, we decided to head for Zhongdian the next day and have an overnight stop in Lijiang. I booked a night for us at the good, small hotel I'd stayed in with Wu Ling and Toshi the previous summer. I knew my friend would appreciate it, just as I had. The six-hour minibus ride was broken only by a stop in a tiny village high up in the mountains. We ate steamed bread and drank Dali beer in a lone wooden hut, surrounded by a family of piglets all eager to gobble up any morsel we should leave.

Lijiang Old Town was as delightful as ever, with its carefree feel and host of smiling faces. The hotel staff greeted me as an old friend and led us to a sunny, clean, comfortable room. We spent that evening in a small café in the ancient market square, taking in all the sights and sounds as we ate wonderful potato croquettes and omelettes. The moon was full and the air super clean, and with virtually no light pollution from street lights, the sky was full of bright stars. In this half-light, we ambled back to our hotel, admiring the sleeping parrots that sat in cages amidst potted plants on front porches.

In Zhongdian, nothing much had changed either. We stayed in a dormitory block of a small guesthouse near the bus station, sharing a room with a Dutch couple on their first visit to China. For them it was the trip of a lifetime, and we sat up half of the night listening to the experiences they'd encountered as they travelled around this enormous country.

The following morning, we ambled around the market areas and local shops and it wasn't long before we found the little boy with the big hairy birthmark on his face. He was still in a tall wicker basket and looked happy and fit. In fact, Mum and Dad also appeared well. I still didn't like what I saw, but at least this family wasn't hungry and who was I to pass judgement?

Taking a taxi to the Guiha Monastery we listened to the maroon-clad novice monks as they played their long wind instruments. The sound, to my untrained ear, was not unlike Rolf Harris's didgeridoo music. Once inside the building we knelt and paid our respects to Buddha and marvelled at the peace and quiet that enveloped us.

"Pity you can't appreciate the fragrances in here," said Judy. "It's a strange mixture of incense and rancid butter, but it's not unpleasant. There's a great feeling of tranquillity, no doubt you can feel it. It's something about all these colours being predominantly red and gold. I love it. There's a lot more to see in this beautiful province and we don't want to run out of time, so let's move on."

We strolled along breathing unpolluted air, passing piles of rocks with prayer flags lying limply between them and slowly made our way back to Zhongdian.

Next day we headed back to Xiaguan, stopping off in Lijiang for one night to enable Judy to look round this beautiful city one more time.

Back in my flat we made preparations for our journey to Jinghong, a city in the Xishuangbanna Dai Autonomous Prefecture, so called because the local people mostly govern themselves. It lies in the deep south of the Province, borders Laos and Myanmar, and has a semi-tropical climate. According to my guidebook it has a distinct Thai feel about it. We would catch a bus from the local bus station and prepare ourselves for a journey that would take anything up to two days to complete. The rainy season had started and nobody knew what hazards lay ahead, as many of the roads would have poor surfaces.

Late afternoon, laden with our rucksacks and bottles of water, we boarded our reasonably clean sleeper bus having booked the double bunk bed behind the driver, something I was later to regret. The drivers, Da Zhang and Fei Li, were preparing for any eventuality and we stared with uncertainty as they loaded spades and pickaxes into the luggage compartments of the bus. We understood they did this trip frequently, so we had to trust these knights of the road. They were cheerful, smiling men in their mid-forties, and although they were talking about us, they gave us a good welcome and helped with our luggage. There was a curtained bed alongside the drivers' seat. One man would be behind the wheel while the other rested, hopefully making this mammoth journey in safety. With a full complement of passengers and the video machine blasting the usual poorly copied tapes which flickered and jumped, Fei Li started the engine. Our trip began to the sound of windows being slammed shut and cigarette lighters clicking into action.

Judy and I sat on our bunk and talked. Our belongings were piled at the foot of the bed, well, at the foot of my half of the bed, because my friend was tall and needed the extra room. We were both excited as we had never been this way before; there would be so much to see, both during the journey and when we got there. Da Zhang, the co-driver, was a friendly guy

251

who could speak a little English and he told us about the villages we passed through.

At eight pm we pulled into a so-called comfort stop as the light was fading. We'd been allocated ten minutes to use the basic facilities and stretch our legs in readiness for the long night ahead. At a snack bar Judy bought a bottle of the local Bai Jiu, better known to me as Chinese whiskey. Back on the bus the lights were switched off, the video player was silent and the smell of sweaty feet began to irritate my friend.

"I'll just have a swig of this sleeping draught", said Judy, winking as she picked up her bottle of spirit. "It'll help me settle and give me a good night's sleep, I hope. She closed her eyes and pulled the grimy grey duvet over her shoulders.

I tried to sleep and was just drifting off when the bus drew to a shuddering halt. We were in a village and all was in darkness. The driver's mate leapt off and I could hear some animated chatter with some women a short distance away. Da Zhang re-appeared accompanied by a young lady and the curtain was hastily drawn round the bed in the front of the bus. Fei Li joined the girl without question, and we were on the road again, with a change of drivers. About this time Judy became restless and started throwing her arms and legs about, squashing me against the restraining rail. There was nothing I could do except try to stop my friend from accidentally pushing me up and over the rail so I sat up. She had no idea of the affects her 'sleeping draught' was having, or what was happening behind the curtain. What could I do except grin and bear it? A restless bed mate was keeping me awake. Sounds of urgent grunting which came from behind the curtained area led me to believe some sort of sex act was taking place only a few yards from my ear. This trip was crazy. Certainly, one for the record, and it had only just begun. I got the distinct feeling this was going to be an interesting few days, to say the least.

At midnight, we pulled into another comfort stop. Although having little sleep I was wide awake and all was silent behind the curtain. I left my sleeping friend and went for a short walk with other passengers. By their expressions they seemed to accept the visiting prostitute as the norm and I said nothing. On my return, the drivers had changed positions. A bleary eyed, but satisfied looking Fei Li was behind the wheel and Da Zhang was missing. I guessed he'd joined the girl. When the muffled noises behind the curtain finally ended, I began to feel drowsy. All around me was quiet and apart from the odd snore, cough and spit everything had returned to normal. With a peaceful Judy by my side I finally fell asleep.

Daylight was breaking as we drew to a halt in something that resembled a huge rain-sodden service station, with fuel pumps, café facilities, and un-manned repair workshops. I must add here that the drivers carried out any maintenance needed on the buses; it was obvious that our knights of the road were men of many talents. After sixteen hours of travelling, cooped up in bunk beds, everyone looked crumpled. We all needed a bit of a wash and a clean-up, and that was all we were going to get in the limited facilities with only an hour allowed. The lady of the night was first to leave. She appeared totally detached by the whole episode and was neat and composed as she hopped off the bus. I thought about her as she melted into the mass of humanity, no doubt she would be searching for her next customer.

Judy and I sat on small stools at low tables and had the usual breakfast of rice-bread twists, crispy deep-fried tofu and bowls of noodles, plus several tumblers of green tea. My friend had not lost her appetite.

"You have no idea of the happenings of last night, have you? You were totally oblivious, and maybe that's fortunate." I laughed and gave a vivid account of the activities. "There is just one thing I ask of you, please don't have any more of your sleeping draught. I just can't cope with it in such a confined space."

"I'm so sorry. I can hardly believe it. Was I really that bad? It must have been a nightmare for you," and with that she emptied the last dregs of the bottle into a puddle at our feet.

Back on board we sat and admired the beautiful scenery as it sped by. "This landscape is so different here," said Judy. "In Guizhou, we have dozens of limestone peaks that are hard to appreciate till you've seen them. In rural areas, we have plots of vegetables, but here, they seem to go for ever or at least as far as the eye can see. Just look at those neat terraces. They go almost to the top of the mountains and are near perfect. It looks as if they've been calculated with a design computer or something."

I smiled, and agreed with every word she said. Without the luxury of air-conditioning, most passengers had their windows open, allowing a flow of air to pass through the bus, so we were fairly comfortable. We passed the hours reading our guidebooks and snoozing on our bunk bed, or watching the mighty Mekong River as it rushed by with no crash barrier or fence between it and the road. As we travelled south, the heat and humidity intensified, as did the rain which reduced our visibility by the hour. At midday, the bus stopped in a small village to re-fuel, a meal for us and a short rest. Squelching through big pools of water we eventually made it to the one and only restaurant. As always, the meal was acceptable. No matter where I was in China, the cooks were always meticulous about their cuisine, even though their choice of dishes was limited because almost everything was produced locally. Fortunately, the rain had eased as we walked the two hundred metre journey on the soggy mud path that led to the communal latrine. The toilets were horrendous with no privacy, we were back to squatting over holes in the dirt floor in a stinking, so Judy said, mud-brick hut. The holes drained into an indescribable open cesspit that joined the ladies and gent's units. You needed a strong stomach to even go near the place, but China offered us no sympathy, nor choice.

"My God, this is awful. It's worse than anything I've come across before. I think it's you who's lucky this time," said Judy. "I won't be able to hold my breath for as long as I would like, but it won't affect you I suppose. You'll never believe what it's like in this heat." I could imagine it. Having a good pair of eyes compensated so often for my loss of sense of smell, and I knew when situations were truly bad. It was an ordeal we both survived.

Back on the bus the rain persisted for the rest of the afternoon, sometimes falling gently and occasionally lashing fiercely against the windscreen. Above us, darkened skies highlighted the electrical storms and non-stop forked lightning which flashed all round us. Our two drivers were sharing only the driving this time, unless of course they fancied another girl! We were glad, as we felt they needed to concentrate on the road ahead, which at times deteriorated to not much more than a gravel track. The swollen river was close to bursting its banks in numerous places. Terrifying to see when we were so near, and unable to do anything except put faith in our knights of the road. Daylight was fading as we approached a right-hand bend and we suddenly came to a juddering halt. The headlights revealed a landslide, a mountain of boulders, mud and slurry which almost enveloped the highway. When the rain eased, the men, including passengers, got busy with spades and pickaxes, while we ladies slowly but surely moved rocks and boulders by hand. After an hour or so, the road was passable and Da Zhang drove our bus until it was clear of the landslide. He shouted, "Walk over now, but be careful." Warily, we passengers found a way through the rock-littered and muddy surface to join him. The river was thundering by only a few metres from us, and in the darkness, this was a scary experience. "This happens from time to time," the driver said "but we are okay and we will get through."

This may not have been a monumental event for the locals, but it was nerve-wracking for us two foreigners, and I wondered if our travelling companions felt the same relief as Judy and I when we reached a proper metalled road. We were grateful to be in one piece and our journey continued in silence.

Finally, we arrived in Jinghong, shattered after our epic journey. Spending so much time squashed up in the bus, our clothes being muddy and sticky we felt as if we'd been travelling for a week. We waved down a bicycle rickshaw and made our way to the Xishuangbanna Guesthouse, a twenty-minute or so ride from the bus terminus. Swaying palm trees lined the dusty roads; partly obscuring the ugly rows of newly built concrete boxes they called hotels. Our guidebooks told us Jinghong was a favourite with Chinese tourists as well as foreigners, because it had a laid-back charm and happy-go-lucky atmosphere. We looked forward to our short break there.

The young receptionist at our hotel looked gorgeous. She had a red flower in her long black hair and wore a white blouse tucked into a short skirt over a black sarong. The wide hems of both skirts were covered in heavy colourful embroidery and the whole outfit looked stunning on her slim body.

We secured a twin-bedded room, lit the mosquito repellent coils, showered in lukewarm water and slept soundly for the next ten hours.

The following morning, we hired bikes and set out to explore the city. In the market area, we sat and enjoyed slices of bananas, oranges, mangoes and kiwis, soaking up the peaceful atmosphere. Life moved at a much slower pace in this part of the world where everyone seemed relaxed as they went about their daily work. At lunch time, we moved on to the National Minorities Park and watched local dancing and singing. There were times I felt I was back in Thailand and wasn't surprised to learn the majority of the population were of Thai origin. Even the local dialect sounded Thai. Most of the people were Buddhists and followed the laws of karma, which gave rise to the calm setting. We loved our few days there.

Two days later we were heading back to my home, travelling this time on Yunnan Airways, not wishing to repeat our journey on the bus. We enjoyed our trip to Jinghong immensely, having met some amazing people who shared not only their way of life, but also their many activities. We were genuinely sorry to leave. Once back in Kunming we updated our diaries and reminisced about our travels to date.

"That terrible bus ride will remain with me forever," mused Judy. "There were times when I really thought we weren't going to make it. But we did, and I guess it's all part of being in this wonderful country that's completely different from everything we've ever known. The way these people look at life is almost beyond my comprehension. I've enjoyed everything about Yunnan so far, now I can't wait to have a quick look at Thailand."

I didn't think I'd forget our few days away together in a hurry, either!

Once in Thailand we planned to spend our time in the north, taking in the city of Chiang Mai and visiting some Hmong tribal people in the rural areas. A return visit to Geoff in his little village on the Laos border was on the cards too, as well as a call on Dr Prakong Vithayasai at the University to arrange her forthcoming visit to Dali for her HIV and AIDS presentation at the medical college.

We landed in Chiang Mai in glorious sunshine and made our way to a guesthouse in the city. I had found this small friendly place on a previous visit and it was well within the city limits, making access easy to all amenities. I had been assured there were no rats in residence, at least none of the four-legged variety. A large ceiling fan kept our room cool and we slept well.

"Why don't we take an elephant ride this morning?" I suggested as we breakfasted, "and this afternoon take a tourist truck out to the Hmong villages. We'll get an air-conditioned bus from Chiang Mai to Ban Kuak tomorrow to see Geoff. He knows we're coming and says we can spend a few days with him. He's had a bungalow built, so accommodation won't be a problem, I hope."

"Sounds fine to me," said Judy. "I'm happy with whatever you plan."

We joined a group of six tourists, four of whom were Japanese. The elephant park was only a short distance out of town. Once in the reserve, these majestic animals seemed as pleased to see us as we were to see them and they nuzzled their soft, warm trunks into our bags for treats, which of course they got. Our elephant was named Tawan. She watched as we climbed the steps of a platform enabling us to reach the seat fixed securely to her back. With her keeper, known as a mahout perched on her neck, she took us on a gentle walk deep into the jungle. Above our heads dozens of monkeys screamed as they leapt from tree to tree, and parrots squawked their shrill replies. We were speechless as Tawan moved gracefully through the rough terrain giving us a truly smooth ride as we listened to the mahout telling us stories. This pair had been together for fifteen years and had spent most of their days hauling enormous logs intended for the furniture trade. Times had changed and sadly trucks and mechanical diggers had taken the place of these gentle giants in the workplace. This whole experience was a real chill-out, something which we both appreciated.

Later, with a guide, we joined a group of Canadian and American tourists and headed north in an old truck in search of the Hmong people on their farms. In a clearing, we came across a cluster of wooden houses built on stilts, with a row of inhabitants waiting to greet us. Obviously, we were expected, and these planned visits possibly provided one or two families with enough extra cash to make some sort of a living. Poverty surrounded us as most people were emaciated and dressed in ragged clothing. There was no electricity and no running water. One family invited us into their single room home, where we saw a baby swinging in a brightly coloured hammock from the rafters above a homemade bed. Giggling, shoeless children of all ages clamoured round for sweets and wanted their photos taken. Some folk, maybe forty-five to fifty years old, which was elderly in that part of the world, lived in separate huts and were smoking pipes full of God knows what.

"There's a very sweet, sickly smell around here," said Judy as our eyes levelled towards the poppies growing in nearby fields. We didn't ask any questions and certainly didn't condemn their habit. It appeared to be the accepted way of life with these gentle people and, after a lifetime toiling away on almost barren plots of parched earth, who would want to change their customs anyway?

Everything was peaceful at the bus station where we queued for our bus tickets to Ban Kuak. The journey would take some four hours, very different from the last time I went, accompanied by Geoff a year ago. He had taken me to so many interesting places en-route, all still very clear in my mind. I would have loved to have taken Judy the same way, but unfortunately there just wasn't time.

Ban Kuak village hadn't changed one bit. The café owner and his wife remembered me from my previous visit, and knew I loved their banana fritters. We tucked into delicious food and drank mugs of hot strong black coffee before walking up the path to Geoff's new bungalow, immediately behind his old house on stilts.

"Peggy", shouted Nit, as she ran towards us. "It's so good to see you again."

Geoff was lying on a sun-bed in the garden. After introductions, all round he told us he'd married Nit, enabling him to buy land to build a bungalow. His back was obviously giving him major problems, and although he could still walk on the level, a flight of stairs was out of the question. I could see he wasn't moving well, but was comfortable and happy with the loving care provided by Nit and her friends.

"I know you don't have much time," said Geoff. "But tomorrow there's a Buddhist funeral, and it's very different from anything you know. I don't think you'll regret the experience. One of my neighbours died today; her family have invited you both to join them for the final goodbye. Obviously, I can't attend so will you go with Nit?"

A funeral wasn't exactly what we'd planned for this visit, but we were curious and wanted to find out what it was all about.

That evening, Nit and a friend took Judy and me on the back of their scooters to her home village. I met the Hmong kids again and some of their families. We sat on the same mud floor in the school room and played with the ragged but beautiful children, their dark eyes shining as they chatted to us in Thai. They'd come a long way since I'd first met them and most were now attending the village school. These children were bright, they worked hard and I hoped they'd have a happy future.

Back at the bungalow, arrangements were being made for supper. Judy and I had bought a dozen bottles of Tiger beer from the local shop, while Nit and three of her friends did the cooking. Geoff sat like a lord in his easy chair. He was obviously enjoying all the attention he was getting from the ladies waiting on him! A clean table cloth had been put on the floor and we sat on cushions in a circle around Geoff. The sticky rice and tasty dips made a great meal and the evening passed very quickly as we all related many stories.

In the morning Nit, Geoff, Judy and I walked to the neighbour's house. Two monks stood either side of an open coffin which had been placed on a wheeled trolley in the courtyard. The casket was surrounded by a polystyrene arrangement that stood two metres high and was fashioned into the most amazing shapes. There were bold swirls, circles, triangles and peaks, all painted in a rainbow of exotic colours. At the head of the coffin, garlands of bright artificial flowers encircled a large photograph of the deceased lady. The relatives were obviously sad, but they believed this lady had gone to a better place. We sat with the family and drank black coffee as a daughter proudly told us about their mother, obviously a very well-loved lady.

At midday, with the monks and close family members to the fore, the cortege was pushed slowly through the village to a designated pyre area about half a kilometre away. Other family members and most of the villagers followed, walking in single file behind the coffin and holding on to a long rope which had been attached to the trolley. Judy, Nit and I tagged on at the end and listened to the chanting of the monks. As we drew near the pyre, Nit led us to a high bank where we could watch the proceedings. The coffin was placed over a large pile of logs which had been stacked between two large concrete struts. Monks chanted and gave blessings to family members. Finally, when everyone was clear, an inflammable liquid was poured over the body and the logs, and the whole thing was ignited. Immediately people started to leave and we followed suit. Some family members would stay until the body was totally cremated. Judy and I hadn't exactly enjoyed the affair, but felt honoured to have been present at a Buddhist village funeral. I'd experienced yet another unforgettable episode.

That afternoon we packed our things and said our farewells to Geoff and Nit. I felt sad at leaving such a vulnerable girl. I wondered what her future would be, and hoped Geoff would look after her. We promised to keep in touch and there were tears as we boarded our bus and set out for the return journey to Chiang Mai.

The next two days were spent exploring the city. Judy loved the night bazaar, seeing people of so many different nationalities and cultures trading together in such peaceful surroundings. Sitting on stools at the roadside we ate hot tasty Thai food, bought too many souvenirs, and soaked up the atmosphere till late into the night.

Next morning, we went to the university where Dr Prakong made us welcome and said she would be more than happy to come to the Medical College in August and would talk about the HIV and AIDS problem in Chiang Mai.

"Will you be able to come here and take me to China with you?" she asked. "I've never been there and you know where you're going. I would appreciate it if you could."

"Yes, I will," I promised. "I'll be in touch as soon as I return to Xiaguan."

It was with a heavy heart that I boarded the Thai Airways flight back to Kunming a few days later. I loved the sense of freedom this country offered every time I visited. China was so different. I often felt inhibited and frustrated, but I only had another six months of my contract to complete and I knew time would fly once I returned to work. Judy and I chatted about our holiday during the flight, agreeing it had been a worthwhile venture. We would meet again at the VSO Conference in Xi'an in November. Arriving at the airport we parted company, Judy to catch her return flight to Guilin, and me heading to the bus station to book a bunk on the night bus back to Xiaguan, where I intended to make arrangements for a short visit to Hiroshima to meet up with my friends Vicky and Ian. We had kept in constant touch since they had left the Teacher's Training College and I was looking forward to seeing them again.

Chapter 40

Vicky and Ian were there to meet me when I landed at Hiroshima Airport. I was delighted they had offered me not only a bed for a few nights, but also a visit to Peace Park as they lived near this eternally monumental piece of land. We spent the first evening deep in conversation as we reminisced and caught up with our news. We were all well and happy and reasonably content with our chosen ways of life. I was delighted to be in their company once more and slept well on their futon that night, but not before experiencing that terrible sinking feeling of isolation and torment I experience whenever I visit a shrine in memory of the dead.

I woke early the next morning excited, but anxious, at the prospect of the promised visit to the renowned Park in the city of Hiroshima where thousands upon thousands of men, women and children were sacrificed in the name of peace on a bright sunny August morning in 1945.

I'd done my research and thought about the atrocities committed by soldiers of all nationalities, including ours, during wartime. Some are worse at it than others and the Japanese certainly excelled in this area. I felt numb when I thought about their horrific deeds in so many parts of the world within my lifetime. It was equally difficult to imagine the scenes all those years ago when this act to end the Second World War took place and the 'Little Boy' the first atom bomb exploded. A huge mushroom shaped cloud blocked everything out, even the sun's rays, and a black, oily rain fell upon a flattened city. It's hard to think about the horror and agonies experienced by survivors, and there were many. Many victims evaporated on the spot, leaving just a shadow on the wall, while others were badly burned or wounded. Those who could run dashed to jump into one of the rivers that ran through the city, but they were burning too, so there was nowhere to go. And worse still, none of the surviving medical teams had any idea how treat such appalling injuries, because no-one had ever experienced anything remotely similar in the past.

But now, as I walked through the gates with my friends the whole place was alive with hundreds of people, mainly Japanese milling around and chatting. Small children were shouting as they scampered and played together. Meanwhile, groups of older children listened intently to their teachers as, I hoped, they learned the reason for the bombing. Dozens of adults were strolling around, whilst others, including monks, were kneeling in prayer and chanting mantras. Flocks of doves flew overhead and damaged trees were beginning to sprout new growth after forty-three years. There was a calm and peaceful atmosphere.

We gazed at a skeletal dome, all which remained of the Prefectural Industrial Hall. This building stands as witness to the destructive power of man and his fearsome nuclear weapon.

I was deep in thought as I reached up to toll the huge Bell of Peace. It was too much to ask for world harmony I knew, but I did my best. Next was a visit to the Peace Memorial Museum where, with dozens of Japanese schoolchildren, we watched a video of the Enola Gay B29 bomber as it took off from America on that fateful day in 1945. We listened to the recorded words of the pilot, Paul Tibbets. The weather and visibility was perfect as he released his cargo. I felt a shudder pass through me.

Afterwards, we sat near the Memorial Cenotaph and watched the Flame of Peace as it flickered in bright sunlight. An inscription beneath stated the blaze wouldn't be extinguished until there were no more nuclear weapons on this earth. Would that ever happen I wondered?

Behind us stood the Children's Peace Monument sitting in a sea of colourful paper cranes. I was mesmerised. Origami is a favourite occupation of Japanese women and girls. There were literally thousands of these paperchains draped on and around the monument that was erected in memory of a little girl named Sadoko Sasaki. She was two years old when the bomb fell and she died of leukaemia when she was twelve. There is an old belief in Japan that a crane can live for a thousand years, and if you can fold a thousand paper cranes you will be protected from illness for ever. I felt very sad when I read this little soul spent many, many hours folding the miniatures when she was sick. She actually managed to make one thousand three hundred cranes. Sadly, it didn't work for her, but before she died she wrote a beautiful poem:

I will write peace
On your wings and you will fly
All over the world.

Directly under the monument are carved these words:

This is our cry;
this is our prayer for building peace in this world.

It was written by a junior high school student.

The multi-coloured paper crane chains were a permanent reminder of the hundreds and hundreds of children who perished at the time of the explosion, and since from its effects. People were still making them to that day.

Fortunately, it seemed the horrendous memories were fading for the inhabitants of Hiroshima, and life was more or less normal. In the few days spent there I found it a pleasant, busy place full of culture, charm and interesting people who were positive and full of hope for the future. The memories of my visit will stay forever.

Chapter 41

And so back to Xiaguan. I'd returned from Japan at six-thirty in the evening. The final leg of the journey was a ride on the night bus from Kunming, always a nightmare because of the on-going road works. I was luckier than most because I could sleep for most of the trip and, although I would feel unwashed, I was usually wide awake at the terminus.

I had a twenty-minute walk in front of me and it was hot and humid. I gazed at a new moon and a lone star that seemed to hover just above the familiar mountain range. It felt good to be home. There were certain idiosyncratic notions I had come to accept with my life in China. I'd learned to curb my curiosity, keep my mouth shut and felt safe.

Night was falling and streets were full of red taxis looking for clients. Their head-lights swept through dust-laden air, revealing crowded pavements. I'd lived in this city for over a year and thought I knew every inch of the area. During my absence road works had taken place, so I found myself trying to find a way around large potholes and confusing pedestrian networks, hindered by extremely poor street lighting. Once in my apartment, I threw down my rucksack, had a shower and slept soundly for eight hours.

In the morning, my first visit was to the post room to pick up my mail. My family and friends hadn't let me down and it was good to get letters from home. I wandered upstairs to my office and was welcomed by the Public Health team, whose facilities I shared. They were the best tea makers in the business and they made sure I was never thirsty or alone for long.

Later, I stood for a few moments outside my bosses' office in the Foreign Affairs Department to report back to work. Would I get a good reception I wondered? I'd been away a month and we had a somewhat strained relationship. I needn't have worried because he was relaxed and smiling as he opened the door. "Sit down," he said. "Have you had a good holiday? Tell me about it sometime. Meanwhile I've got some good news for you. You've been awarded a medal from the Governor of the Province for your efforts in raising awareness of HIV and AIDS. He knows of the work you've done and he's delighted. Only five awards of this nature are awarded annually and they're presented to foreigners who work here in Yunnan. We're very proud of you; congratulations, Peggy. The Governor, Mr Li, will come to Kunming and make the presentation sometime in September. When I know more I'll tell you. This is a real honour, not only for you, but for the college as well. Well done." There was no sarcasm in his voice and his tone was very genial.

I sat down, hardly able to believe what I had heard. But it was true and I knew my stubbornness and tenacity had been worth every minute.

"David, that's brilliant. What a wonderful surprise." I gulped with excitement having never heard of such an award in China, let alone considered the possibility of receiving one.

"I'm so pleased to be back and with your help I hope to be able to continue this work for the rest of my time here. While we are on the subject of HIV and AIDS, I spent time with Dr Prakong Vithayasai in Chiang Mai University when I was in Thailand, and she is happy to come and give a two-day presentation on her experience in her city. August 28th and 29th are good dates for her. I know we've discussed this before, and I'm certain we'll all benefit from her knowledge, especially the doctors. She will bring information on courses they hold at the university with her. Your doctors will be very welcome to attend them."

"Good. That's excellent. I'll make all the necessary arrangements. Just let me know what she needs." With his words ringing in my ears I left the office.

I was walking on air as I made my way back to my flat. Rumei would be the first to hear my good news about the award. Part of me felt she should be getting one as well because I couldn't have done much without her. She'd been such a good friend. We trusted each other implicitly and together we had made this achievement possible.

But now it was back to work. I sent a fax to Dr Prakong in Thailand, requesting a programme for her visit. There were less than two weeks to prepare and I wanted everything to be perfect for this distinguished lady. The Foreign Affairs Department had given me permission to leave the country on August 23rd and return on the 28th with Dr Prakong. They would deal with my exit and re-entry visas and the college vehicle would pick us up from the airport. The doctor would stay at a hotel near the college. At her request, the first presentation was to take place before a small group of college leaders, cadres or party bosses, clinical teachers and some medical personnel. The second, on the following day, would be presented to the rest of the college staff, including as many students as we could cram into the building. No health and safety rules here. The doctor would use English as the common language and the official college translator would be at her disposal.

The next few days flew by, and almost before I knew it I was heading back to Kunming on the night bus in readiness for my flight to Thailand. I loved the whole journey. I was having an unscheduled break and looked forward to seeing the smiling Thai people again. I would have four full days in my favourite guest house, the Pathara in Moonmuang Road, before joining Dr Prakong for the journey back to Xiaguan.

It was hot and stuffy in Chiang Mai and the mosquitoes gave me hell, but I didn't mind too much and liberally applied the anti-bite cream to all exposed areas. I loved the free and easy atmosphere in and around the city and enjoyed the company of new friends at the guesthouse.

On the flight to Kunming Dr Prakong and I discussed the schedule for her presentations. I was able to assure her that her requirements had been met at the college and everyone was keen to learn from her experiences. David had guaranteed a room reservation in the nearby hotel.

Charles, from the Foreign Affairs Department and good old 007, the college driver, were at the airport to meet us. The four-hundred-kilometre drive would take the usual fifteen hours or so to complete but we would be comfortable in the four-wheel drive. In due course, we pulled into a roadside café for refreshments.

"I need the bathroom," whispered Dr Prakong. "Will you show me where it is please? As a Thai, I can't read these funny Chinese characters."

"Of course, I will. I need one as well. Follow me." I said with a terrible sinking feeling. I'd been to this particular set of holes in the hard mud floor before. They were awful. I tried to warn my friend, this lovely lady who was accustomed to tiled, spotless flush toilets, but found it difficult to explain. She was appalled when she saw it, but in the end, as there was no option, she tied her scarf tightly around her mouth and nose, took a deep breath and went for it.

"I don't ever want to go anywhere like that again," she exclaimed as we searched for a hosepipe outside the café to wash our hands. "It was terrible. How on earth do you cope?"

274

"When you have no alternative, you have to. But I'll never get used to it." I replied with a wry smile and took her arm. "That's how it is in some places, but things are getting better, honestly."

The rest of the journey was uneventful and we arrived at the Medical College in the early hours of the morning. My boss was waiting for us and after introductions we headed to a college dining room for a late supper, or perhaps an early breakfast.

"Peggy, there's been a slight change in the arrangements. Everything regarding Dr Prakong's lectures is fine. The hall is prepared and the college interpreter will act for her. But, because I was unable to book a room in the nearby hotel our guest will have to stay with you. Will that be OK?"

What choice did I have? I didn't feel it was quite the right thing for the lady to have to bed-down in my scruffy flat. Fortunately, we got on very well and I hoped she would be comfortable. That night I gave up my cosy bed and room and settled for an uncomfortable night in my spare room. I slept on a flimsy flock mattress covering the solid wooden structure they called a bed.

Next day, after we had lingered over breakfast in a nearby eatery I took Dr Prakong for a tour of the college. Although the whole place looked grimy and grey, with some of the two thousand students milling around I felt it had a well-worn homely feel about it. My visitor passed no comment and I wondered how she viewed this establishment. After all, Chiang

Mai University Hospital was a gleaming white, fairly modern building. There were plenty of students in Thailand, but they didn't live in such close proximity and their campus had an air of orderly activity.

At two o'clock we made our way to the lecture hall. The twenty-five specially invited college leaders, cadres, clinical teachers and senior medical personnel were seated at the front of the hall. Most were middle-aged men with expressionless faces. I hardly knew any of them. As Dr Prakong took her place at the podium, I sat with Rumei at a table at the side of the stage, in case assistance was required by the interpreter. The pale-faced girl looked apprehensive but she was ready and the lecture began.

"Do you know the most common transmission route for HIV?" she asked the audience. After a pause she continued, "Its sex, unprotected sex."

She repeated this message to each member of the audience pointing to them, one by one.

"Sex, sex and more sex. Different kinds of sex with no protection. That is how most people in the world have become infected with this terrible disease. It is not always their fault. How can they be to blame when nobody has told them about it? They simply didn't know the dangers and prostitution is the world's oldest profession."

The poor interpreter struggled, not with the translation because her English was near perfect, but with the content. You just didn't say the word sex; it was as simple as that. Dr

Prakong was not put off. In fact, I think she rather enjoyed the looks of horror that appeared on the majority of faces as she told them she didn't think Chinese men in the audience were any different from Thai men, or any other men throughout the world.

As the lecture continued, the poor interpreter stuttered and became so embarrassed she eventually ran off stage. Rumei had to take over and as always coped magnificently. Nothing fazed that girl.

I sat at my desk. What had I done? I had organised this visit and felt an acute sense of responsibility, but how could I be to blame? Little did I realise the doctor would start her presentation in such an explicit way. I always approached the subject in a gentler manner, because I had learned to manage these audiences through trial and error, but this was out of my control. I tried to make myself as small as possible, wanting to slide beneath my desk. I wondered what the reaction would be at the end of the day, to what could only be described as a provocative session to a culturally prudent and conservative audience. Would I still have a job in this strange and intriguing land tomorrow, I asked myself?

The session progressed with the doctor explaining how she and her paediatrician husband initially became involved with the epidemic in Chang Mai, when several babies with HIV were abandoned on the wards. They had come to realise a terrible thing was happening on their very doorstep and set about doing something positive about it. Together they visited many of the parlours, night clubs, brothels and other places where people met. They wanted everybody to understand the dangers of unprotected sex and intravenous drug use. Information leaflets in ordinary everyday language were posted just about everywhere in the city, also hot-line telephones were installed. They aimed to get one hundred percent usage of condoms, but doubted this aspiration would ever be achievable.

The audience sat and listened. I would never know what went through the minds of those college leaders and cadres. Dr Prakong had made some strong, clear statements and I could only hope they had taken it on board. In my area, there were no information leaflets or posters that I could see, but perhaps I was still looking in the wrong places.

The session came to an end and the audience left the building. The Doctor and I went back to my flat. She needed a strong cup of coffee and a good chat.

The following day brought no repercussions and I breathed a huge sigh of relief. I didn't want anything to upset Dr Prakong's visit. She had given valuable time and effort. After breakfast, I was overjoyed when an audience of over three hundred doctors, senior nurses and students from the college and nearby hospitals arrived for the morning's presentation. Rumei was on hand to translate and the sessions flowed with her knowledge and ability. She'd never been to Chiang Mai, but I'd given her as much information as I could, and as always, she knew how to get the message over to her own people. The morning flew by and soon it was time to bring the two-day meeting to a close. At a special lunch, the doctor was thanked by the college hierarchy. David, my boss, spoke highly of the event, thanking me for bringing Dr Prakong to the college, and for the introduction to Chiang Mai University, which the college hoped to utilise sometime in the future for doctor training in HIV and AIDS.

That afternoon the doctor and I flew from Dali to Kunming, where she would fly home to Thailand. At the airport, I thanked her for coming and giving up her valuable time to give such excellent lectures.

"It's what I do," she said, "and I've enjoyed staying with you. It might not have been the finest apartment, but we got on well and had many laughs."

It was true, we had blended well and she was good company. I had developed a great respect for this lady, finding her both inspiring and stimulating. I promised to visit her and the orphans in their homes on my next visit to Chiang Mai, which I hoped would be in the not too distant future.

Chapter 42

Adrenaline was flowing freely as I stood outside the large white double doors that led to a conference room at the Green Dragon Hotel in Kunming. The date was the 29th September, the day for the presentation of the Friendship with Yunnan Awards. The dress code for the occasion was formal, and the only frock I possessed at that time was a well-worn blue denim one. Thank God for good old Marks and Spencer's I thought as I took the early flight from Dali. The outfit wasn't terribly smart, but looked good and I hoped it would be acceptable. In the coffee lounge, I met up with my programme officer from Beijing and the four other recipients. I was delighted to discover that John, the VSO teacher from Kunming who I had met the previous year, was to get an award as was another Englishman and two Dutchmen. We stood in a little group and chatted nervously, with none of us knowing what to expect when the doors opened. I didn't have long to wait.

"Margaret Barnes. Come please?" A petite Chinese woman appeared and took me by the arm. "Follow me," she said.

As we walked through the doorway my knees were knocking. I was immediately confronted by a neat line of Chinese politicians all seemingly sporting the same sleeked black hair styles, black suits with gleaming white shirts, red ties and shiny black shoes. Mr Li, the Governor of the Province stepped forward and, as he shook my hand, he said through his interpreter, "Margaret Barnes. I award you this Certificate and Medal of Friendship with Yunnan in appreciation of your enthusiastic support and friendly co-operation in the construction undertakings of Yunnan Province in the People's Republic of China." He smiled as he hung the heavy medal around my neck and presented me with a certificate.

"Thank you. I'm very happy to be here. This award is not only for me and VSO, but also for my professional colleagues at the Medical College and all the people who have helped and supported me. Thank you so very much." And at that moment I knew I couldn't have any better permission to continue my expanding role at the Medical College!

I was moved along the line to meet and shake hands with other dignitaries. Out of the corner of my eye I saw the next recipient being ushered in. Thank goodness that's over I thought to myself as I looked around. There were twelve neatly arranged dark brown leather armchairs, each one with cream lacy antimacassars on the arms and headrests. I hadn't seen coverings like that since childhood, when visiting my grandparents, and a smile crossed my face. Small tables, heaped with tall vases of colourful flowers sat at the side of each chair. I was reminded of pictures I'd seen on TV of sober faced Chinese politicians sitting in a row and now it looked as if I was about to join them. I never thought this would ever happen to me and I continued smiling as I was led to my seat.

After the presentations and the long-winded speeches that followed, Mr Li sat next to me. With the help of an interpreter my jagged nerves were finally laid to rest and we chatted amiably.

Afterwards, we attended a lavish dinner party at the hotel with the dignitaries. Alcohol flowed and we dined from gold-painted bowls with gold-coloured chopsticks. The food was delicious and included assorted fried vegetables, sautéed beef slices with black pepper sauce, braised chicken and steamed buckwheat buns with Yunnan ham. Deep-fried fish cubes and egg-fried rice completed the first course. So, this was how the other half lived! Much later, after ice-cream and coffee, we five medal winners left for our respective hotels knowing we'd had yet another extraordinary day to remember.

Chapter 43

I kept in constant touch with the VSO office in Beijing, to keep them aware of my changing role. This was new ground for one of its volunteers and it was an extremely sensitive issue. An HIV and AIDS team had been formed at the college. The members being myself, David, my boss, the two doctors who had created the outreach clinic in the city, and Professor Yang Ting Shi, head of the Public Health Department. We met at regular intervals and discussed our progress on the educational front. Meanwhile, I applied for an extension to my placement. I hadn't originally come to teach prevention of HIV; my role had just evolved and I had discovered a need which was so important to the local community. I wanted to continue, but that decision wasn't up to me. I'd have to be patient.

I sat enjoying cups of green tea and the warm sunshine in front of my favourite restaurant near the medical college. I watched the usual menagerie of chickens, frogs and fish and waited for Simon Johnson to arrive. I'd received faxes from VSO and the British Embassy telling me that he was taking another short break in Dali and wanted to see how the clinic in Xiaguan was progressing. I was not only looking forward to this work-related visit, but also catching up on what was going on in the world. There was much to tell him about our college project, and I wondered what his response would be. We desperately needed money, and that didn't come within the proviso of VSO; they provided volunteers only, hoping a little of their teaching expertise and skills would remain after returning home.

Quite suddenly I saw him walking towards me. After a friendly greeting, I ordered more tea and we got down to business. I said to him "I'll ring David and tell him you're here. He's going to meet us at the clinic, so, when you're ready we'll take a taxi."

Once in the clinic, Simon looked at me and said "I can see nothing much has changed here since my last visit. The whole clinic is clean and tidy, but unfortunately, the only tap for running water is still in the squat latrine on the ground floor. I'll make a note of this," as he wrote the information on a pad. We toured the whole building, with my visitor making many notes as he chatted to David, me and the two doctors who had created the clinic.

That evening, Simon told me about a grant which might be available from the Global Issues Command. This organisation, within the British Government, provides insight into global events based on sustainability. The Foreign and Commonwealth Office in Beijing were able to apply for the funding, but a proposal would have to be submitted. The grant would have to be used in the six months following its approval. Simon and I sat up half the night, sipping Dali beer and making notes before a plan was produced. This included the training of health care workers, teachers, barefoot doctors who practised in rural villages, local children and prostitutes in AIDS prevention and education. We would design education and training materials and provide information packs, targeting the above groups. All this would be in conjunction with the Dali Health Bureau. An HIV and AIDS specialist would be invited to speak at the college with all the costs being met. Upgrading of the outreach clinic would be included, and a project would place throughout the Dali Prefecture to discover what the local population knew about HIV. The grand total would amount to ten thousand British Pounds. When converted to the Chinese currency, the Yuan, it was an awful lot of money. I decided I'd start to worry about that if, and when, the award was made and we discussed the formalities as far as possible. I was tired, but couldn't help feeling the ripple of excitement that almost overwhelmed me with the prospect of staying on in this beautiful neighbourhood for another year. I had grown to love it and getting this much-needed project off the ground was important to me. I was delighted that Simon had taken such an interest in our early plans at the college. Without his input, I would have been packing my belongings and heading for repatriation in a few weeks' time. But now, hopefully, I would be able to stay in my beloved Dali and move forward.

Much later, after seeing Simon off in a taxi, I crawled into my bed with the events of the evening racing around in my head. It wasn't going to be a 'walk over'. At times, the local political issues nearly drove me mad. But equally, I knew what

I was capable of, and felt the contents in the proposal were well within my reach. Of course, I would have to await the outcome, but I felt positive and could visualise yet another challenge on the horizon.

Early next morning, I was in the Foreign Affairs office to talk to my boss. He was overjoyed at the news and promised to do all he could to help. I telephoned the VSO office in Beijing to keep them updated with the proposal that Simon Johnson was going to make to the British Government. It was essential they knew what was going on. The annual VSO conference was due to take place in Xian the following week, and I had been given a slot to talk about the HIV and AIDS problem in the Yunnan area to my peers. The conference would provide an opportunity to talk over Simon's proposal with the project officers and allow me to discuss the possibility of an extension to my placement within the Province. I knew Simon would be in touch with them to provide the details, but I needed their approval for my peace of mind.

The next few days slipped by, and almost before I knew it I was settled once again on the night bus heading for Kunming. I was looking forward to meeting up with my VSO teacher colleagues, and making the flight with them to the annual conference in Xian. I had perfected my presentation, which would take place on the second day. It was neatly packed inside my rucksack. Lulled into a deep sleep with the combination of smoke laden air, the constant crack of sun flower seeds being split, and the sound of soft snoring from my neighbour, I fell asleep.

I was rudely awakened by an amplified, tinny shrieking noise. It was about two o'clock in the morning and we had pulled into a filling station, not only to refuel, but also to take advantage of the comfort stop. I looked up and watched as three extremely thin men were boarding the bus. Through a loud hailer they ordered us to get off and leave all bags behind. They were the dreaded armed security police, wearing oversized green uniforms with peaked caps that looked far too big for their seemingly small heads. Sadly, they lacked the physical presence for the job, in my opinion anyway. I watched as my fellow travellers shook themselves awake, jumping to their feet before stumbling off the bus. I followed knowing better than to argue with the law.

"What on earth is going on," I thought to myself as I joined the motley, bedraggled group on the tarmac. I soon found out, as I watched the men move up and down the coach opening bags and boxes. I became anxious, wondering if the driver might move his vehicle. There were possibly twenty almost identical coaches neatly parked in straight lines nearby, all going through the same rigmarole. I stood at the front of my bus and leaned against the bonnet, determined not to lose the sight or feel of my precious transport. Finally, after about half an hour we were allowed to re-board. I could see a cursory check of my belongings had taken place, but nothing had been tampered with.

This search treatment was new to me, but I was well aware of the drug problems in the province and guessed these security men were only doing what they were paid for. On subsequent bus trips I learned to lie still and feign sleep. There were always a few mutterings about the *'Lao Wei,'* or foreigner, but at least they left me alone, possibly because they couldn't speak English.

The VSO conference was a welcome relief from the stresses of life that came with living and working in a foreign country. As before, it was good to get with the now somewhat diminished group of volunteers I had originally travelled with from the United Kingdom. During the days, we attended talks and chatted to our programme officers. In the evenings, we crowded around the bars, drinking too much beer, and renewing acquaintances as we re-lived experiences, good and bad, generally letting off steam. My HIV and AIDS session was well received; I had given a presentation that had provided much food for thought for my one hundred or so VSO colleagues. They had responded with enthusiasm. I was very pleased and knew I'd done well. I now looked forward to returning to the Medical College in a couple of days to continue my work. Whether or not I would be granted an extension to my placement, I still didn't know.

Chapter 44

On his visit a few weeks before, Simon had mentioned World AIDS Day on December 1st, this was a special day and I had taken it up with my boss.

"If you can get something organised I'll support you," he said. "I'll arrange a meeting with the Dali Health Bureau and the Anti-epidemic Centre. Our Public Health Team will be heavily involved as well. See what you can come up with and let me know."

The meeting with the teams went well, with everyone accepting my staging and presentation ideas. We were all keen to make this first ever public exhibition on HIV and AIDS a genuine success in the city. It was unanimously agreed that the information should be simple and basic, helped by colourful posters and the spoken word. The local radio and television teams were to take part, and would provide a huge boost to our efforts.

"I know we have very little money at our disposal, so I will make a contribution to cover the cost of simple information leaflets as long as they will be understood by everyone, both the educated and the not so well-informed members of the general public." I told them.

I worked with the Public Health team to produce a simple but comprehensive leaflet. I remembered the terrible error made in the UK in the 1980's, when every household had blue printed information leaflets slipped through all letter boxes. It had contained all the information the government thought we, the general public, should know about HIV and AIDS. Unfortunately, they didn't realise that most people couldn't understand the technical language and threw the pamphlet away. This blunder cost the country a considerable amount of money as the information had to be re-issued with the use of everyday language. I didn't want the same to happen here.

There couldn't have been much narrow red ribbon left in the local shops after I had bought hundreds of metres of the stuff, together with dozens of boxes of pins. My student friends quickly learned how to make red ribbon emblems. Within a week of my request nearly four thousand ribbons had been carefully folded, pinned and delivered to my office. They were proud of their achievement and were glad to have been able to play a part, no matter how small.

With the weather being warm and dry, the wide pavement on a busy street in the centre of Xiaguan was swarming with inquisitive onlookers. The Public health team had made informative posters, also a huge colourful banner with the words Force for Change – World AIDS Campaign with Young People in bold red letters, both in English and Chinese. The banner itself brought people to a standstill as they read and digested the information. Being practical and business-like, I needed to be among the people, whereas my Chinese counterparts were shy and retiring, and sat behind their six decorated tables. They did a tremendous amount of teaching that day though, as they handed out leaflets and explained what the presentation was all about. I was busy mixing with the crowd, pinning red ribbons on collars, lapels and shirts and pushing information packs into their hands. The TV crews interviewed the heads of the Public Health team, the Anti-epidemic Centre and me.

At the end of the day, a group of friends gathered in my flat to watch the local television news. Big cheers went up when they saw me as the celebrity of the moment.

It was good to know our efforts had been successful, and obviously appreciated by so many ordinary people with their comments on the programme.

Chapter 45

A few days later I felt on top of the world and thought that maybe there was someone up there looking down on me after all? Earlier in the day I had been summoned to the fax room. Climbing the stairs to his office, I could hear my friend Mr Ma whistling a snappy tune. I liked this man and we had a good relationship

"Ahhh, Peggy," he said. "You have fux. No, two fux today. Would you like tea with me? I show you picture of my daughter."

We sat together and sipped green tea. I admired his family snapshots. His pretty daughter had graduated from university a few months earlier; he was a very proud and happy father.

"Beautiful." I said. "She's a lovely girl and you're a lucky man."

Finally, I could read my faxes which gave me the brilliant news from both VSO and Simon Johnson from the British Embassy. I'd been granted a year's extension to my placement and would be sponsored by Martin Gordon OBE of the Barry and Martin's Trust. This was the organisation which had funded the workshops I'd organised and taken part in. I was delighted and equally thrilled to learn that the grant of almost ten thousand British Pounds from the Global Issues Command had been approved. This would facilitate our planned local project of awareness and education of HIV and AIDS in the west of Yunnan province. The logistics of this large sum of money would take place in the New Year. Details of the operation made me feel somewhat nervous, but the ever-present optimism in me knew it would be sorted out when the time was right. I was so happy I could have kissed the messenger, but instead went to have a chat with my boss. Outwardly he was delighted at the news. Now aware of the extent of the HIV and AIDS problem surrounding us, he knew help was needed. What he actually felt about having to put up with me for another year I would never know, as we often disagreed and argued, but he assured me my flat would be made available for as long as I needed it.

A meeting of our HIV and AIDS team was arranged. A managerial team was formed and would run alongside the working panel. I was included in both. My colleagues would select a local bank to hold the money. Any cheque would require three signatures from the managerial team, including me, prior to any withdrawals. A fax from Simon informed us that the first joint venture with a condom company in Shandong Province had been set up. This would benefit the population and maybe colourful 'johnnies' would appear in the local clinics, or maybe not, depending on the thoughts of the local health officials. I was delighted, but there was muted reaction from my colleagues. Eventually, contracts were signed and returned to the Embassy and VSO.

I contacted VSO and spoke to my programme officer. There was a policy within this organisation, which allowed volunteers to return to their home country for one month with full expenses paid if they extended the contract. As I lived so near to Thailand I would be able to fly from Bangkok.

Two days later, I received an email from Martin Gordon inviting me to visit him at his London home during my UK break. It would be a pleasure to meet the mystery man who had funded our HIV and AIDS workshops. I would also be able to meet up with Fiona and Penny, the head nurse and doctor from the Chelsea and Westminster Hospital. These lovely people had provided me with much needed literature, and given me the support and confidence I needed to continue my role at that time.

As I made preparations for my journey home, I thought about the last two years of my life. Meeting Vicky and Ian, the English teachers from Australia was the best thing that could have happened to me. They had taught me all they knew about China, its people and their way of life, drawing on their eight years' experience of teaching and living in different parts of the country. I don't think I would have survived the first six months without their concern and encouragement,

The term was almost at its close. I kept myself busy teaching the doctors in the evenings, and studying my books on HIV and AIDS. I spent time in Dali with Jianbuo, Jack and Stella in Jack's Café. I seemed to have known these three people forever. They had been good friends, and I appreciated their kindness and hospitality in an otherwise alien country. Christmas was fast approaching and I'd decided to spend it in Thailand, relaxing with friends. I knew I'd have to return to the Medical College to attend meetings before I could fly home, but I felt I needed a few days away from China. Prior to my departure I secured my exit and re-entry visas and was then ready to go.

Reaching Chiang Mai in Thailand on Christmas Eve, I made my way to the guesthouse in Moon Muang Road. That evening I wandered down to the local drinking house used by several expatriate English rugby club types with their wives and girlfriends. I loved linking up with these individuals and making new acquaintances. It was a little piece of England and they always included me in their group. Christmas and New Year in their company was great fun. In between celebrations, I managed a couple of amazing elephant rides and a cruise on the River Ping. I also secured my ticket for my journey to England in the middle of January and some small gifts for my family and friends.

I returned to China for a few days to attend meetings, and finally I was on my way home.

Chapter 46

I drifted in and out of sleep on the Thai Airways jumbo on the night flight from Bangkok to London's Heathrow airport, thinking about my four-week break in England. Apart from catching up on news from family and friends, I needed to organize a trip to London to visit Martin Gordon and Fiona and Penny. Martin had invited me to his home to meet him and some of the donors for the Barry and Martin's Trust. Fiona, one of the British speakers at the first HIV and AIDS workshop in Kunming, had suggested I spend a day at the Kobler Clinic at the Chelsea and Westminster Hospital, and I was keen to take up this opportunity. But for the most part I was thinking about my family and friends. Having been away for two years I knew I'd changed; not only in my physical appearance because of my weight loss, but also in my view on life and living. I'd undergone some humbling experiences in the last two years and my long-term outlook had completely changed. Material things were no longer important; my values had almost become those of the developing nations, where, as long as I was warm, had enough sleep and wasn't hungry, I was fine. My grandchildren, Jack, Max, Rufus and Dillon would be two years older, and surely have grown in many ways. Would they have developed the typical western attitudes, where the right label on jeans and trainers was vital to the modern schoolboy? I'd soon find out. My youngest son Mike and his wife Lu had a new baby, Archie, born in November. I could hardly wait to see them all.

Nearly twelve hours after take-off, the jumbo drew to a halt. I was so excited I could hardly wait to disembark even though it was a cold, wet, miserable morning. I didn't care; I was back in England and wanted to land both feet on British soil once more. The adrenaline was flowing as I stood in the gangway of the plane. Once in the airport I waited impatiently for my rucksack to appear on the conveyor belt. Then, quite suddenly, I was in the arms of my family. I was home at last.

The following four weeks passed in a blissful blur; a fuzz of joyful family parties and reunions. It was a sheer delight to see friends and relatives who had written the welcomed letters with snippets of news from all over the UK. Many had sent little gifts that meant so much and kept me going when I had my 'low' moments.

I enjoyed beautiful English roast dinners, such as roast beef and Yorkshire pudding. I had thought about this type of food frequently during the last two years, it was a welcome change from noodle soup. Sometimes I ate too much and felt quite poorly, but was happy to do so because I didn't want to miss anything good on the table.

I thoroughly enjoyed the delightful task of getting to know my grandchildren again. They sat spellbound as I reeled off tales of my life in a strange and foreign land. I told them about the children I knew, how they lived and what they learned at school. I met long-term friends in favourite bars. We laughed and reminisced, drinking John Smith's bitter and eating pub-grub. My dear friend Margaret took me shopping for items I couldn't find in Xiaguan, things like cotton knickers, and socks. Birds' custard powder, jelly cubes, Marmite, Bovril and stock cubes were also on the list because sometimes it felt good to know what I was eating, even though I was rarely ill in China.

I'd missed my home country a great deal, and remembered most of our public places as being fairly quiet and organised. It's strange how one's mind plays tricks from time to time, as I discovered when I queued in the local Post Office. I stood in what I can only describe as an excuse for a queue, listening to the whingeing and grumbling I had completely forgotten about. I was quite glad to buy my stamps and leave.

I was in for a shock when I plucked up the courage to do the weekly shop at Tesco's Supermarket alone. In the toiletries department, I gazed at the assortment and colours of the toilet rolls on display. I could get loo rolls in Xiaguan, but they were all white and had the trade name of 'White Cat' boldly displayed on them. It was the same with the dishwashing liquid and soap powder, all in the identical bland packaging of the 'White Cat' company. I stood and listened in disbelief as a young couple pontificated and argued over which coloured toilet roll matched their bathroom suite! At that point, I'd had enough and left the store. It was then I knew that the immense cultural differences I'd experienced had affected me deeply.

My trip to London was inspirational. An enjoyable evening was spent with Martin Gordon at his home. I gave a short talk on my work in China to a group of donors of the Barry and Martin's Trust. My presentation was well received by this remarkable group of delightful individuals. Martin explained how the Trust had come into being a short time after Barry's untimely death from AIDS and I felt proud to be included, and even more determined to continue my work in China.

The next day brought the promised visit to The Kobler Clinic at The Chelsea and Westminster Hospital with Fiona Gracie, the head Nurse at this HIV clinic, the largest of its kind in The United Kingdom at that time. In the outpatients department, I spoke to patients and relatives and friends in an informal atmosphere that was both enlightening and positive. Visiting a ward, I was humbled as I listened to a seriously ill man who was so at ease with me. I could have stayed with him for hours, but eventually had to leave.

All too soon I had to say said goodbye to family and friends and set off for Heathrow Airport again. This time I was laden with little English gifts for my Chinese friends and looking forward to my return to China.

Chapter 47

The journey to Kunming from London was exhausting. All I wanted to do was collapse on to nice comfy bed in the room I'd previously booked at the Camellia Hotel. I loved this place; it was my last hope of pure relaxation before starting on the endless trip to Xiaguan on the grubby night-sleeper bus in four days' time.

"Peggy. What are you doing here?" A breathless Jo ran towards me as I was about to enter the hotel. "I'm on my way home to celebrate our New Year, and I'd love you to come with me."

Jo, a nursing degree student from Dali Medical College not only had an excitable and bubbly persona, but also a near perfect command of the English language. I liked and admired her for her positive attitude.

"It sounds wonderful Jo, but let's go inside first and talk about it. I desperately need a drink of some kind and a five-minute rest before I do anything".

Once seated at the bar, I sipped a Coke and listened.

"Jiaquan Ge, one of my cousins will pick us up in his car and take us to his village called Hong Xi, or Rainbow Brook," she said. "It's my Dad's hometown and where his brother lives with his family. This is a very special time for us, because all Chinese families like to spend this holiday together."

I knew these people loved to celebrate their New Year like nobody else. I'd enjoyed previous New Year activities, but this excursion promised to be different as I would be heading off to the South of Yunnan Province to a very small village and would be with a family. This was an opportunity I didn't want to miss. I knew the Foreign Affairs Department at the Medical College would frown upon my judgement; visiting students' homes was not encouraged. There was always the safety aspect, but I felt secure with this girl at my side and, what the hell, I'd made my choice, I was going.

"Jo, it sounds wonderful. Thank you very much. I will come, but first let me cancel my room and put my luggage into storage. I'll be ready when I've put a few things together," I left her making a phone call to her cousin, and nipped out to buy a bottle of Bai Jiu, the Chinese whiskey, for the celebration.

Five hours later, just after midnight, we arrived in Hong Xi village. My tiredness had disappeared as I stood on the dirt lane and stretched my legs. The silence was deafening. The air was warm and dry; above us was a cloudless sky with a new moon surrounded by hundreds of twinkling stars. Slowly I grew used to the dim light and could see the shapes of dwellings nearby. Jo and her cousin led me to a house where, after being introduced to her father and his brother's family, a feast of rice, fish, and vegetables awaited me. Eventually I was taken to a bedroom by torchlight where I soon fell into a deep sleep, knowing I'd have to wait until morning to see exactly where I was.

The mud-walled house was quite big by Chinese standards. A large living room in the centre had a bedroom leading off each corner. There were three more rooms upstairs which were used for grain storage, plus general household commodities. The kitchen was large and contained an enormous wok on a briquette stove, a couple of buckets of water, a pile of vegetables, a long hosepipe with a tap attached and a low table with plenty of stools around. In one corner, a sunken concrete square with a hole in a corner acted as a drain. Part of the roof was open, planned this way because of the constant heat in that part of the world. There was no bathroom of course, but across the yard there was a typical squat latrine, with two planks secured over a hole. Some privacy was provided by a couple of straggly bushes!

In daylight, I could begin to appreciate just where I was and get to know the family. Apart from Jo, there was her father, his brother and son, wife, plus their three children. Jinquan Ge, the car driver, was nineteen, a pretty daughter was sixteen and the younger son was twelve. The second and third child, much loved additions, had cost the family a hefty fine paid to local government officials. They were a very happy, friendly group and as Jo was the first member of the family to go to college, they were obviously proud of her. My family photos created great interest as none of them had ever seen children with blond hair and blue eyes before. Tonight, we would all be celebrating the Chinese New Year, when Chinese families get together, celebrate and have great fun. I felt fortunate to be included as my own family were so far away.

The village was small and pretty, consisting of twenty or thirty houses, all constructed of mud brick. A junior school for seven to eleven-year olds stood in the centre with a dormitory attached. It was not unusual in country areas for children from the outlying villages to board from Monday to Friday, or even for the whole term if their families were so poor they were unable to provide money for travelling. The secondary school was in the nearest large town, again with boarding facilities. The village stood on the top of a hill and was surrounded by valleys with the usual neat lines of cabbages, tobacco and grain. A short distance beyond them was a mountain range with a bluish pink hue, the peaks melting into fluffy white clouds. In a large muddy water hole, a woman was leading a buffalo on a piece of string. They were both up to their knees in water. Other women were spreading cabbage leaves out to dry until ready for pickling and eating at a later date. A short distance away was a deep well providing clean water. I felt quite safe with this, because no matter where I went in China the water was always boiled and drinkable, something which I appreciated. The scantily clad local kids greeted me with the usual "Ello". They looked healthy and happy, running around on bare feet, oblivious of the stones and pebbles, just as I did when I was small. Their parents were poor peasant farmers who obviously cared for their children. There were no fridges here and the people managed in the same way as they had done for hundreds of years, as my family did during my childhood. The soil was very dry and crumbly and the crops looked spindly and sparse because it hadn't rained in five months. The rice season had just ended and the resulting straw was piled high around the village. This would be used for weaving into sleeping mats or animal bedding.

"Come on," said Jo as she took my arm. "Let's go for a walk. I want to show you some interesting places; it's too good to be staying in."

As we strolled towards the sparkling waters of a large lake, I stood and watched a man guiding two water buffaloes as they slowly dragged the homemade plough over the packed soil. These beautiful animals were extremely placid, spending most of their lives with humans, probably sleeping in a shed a few yards from their owners. It was a bit sad knowing they were to be killed and eaten at the end of their working lives, but that's economics for you, and pretty tough meat at the end of the day! A few old men sat around the shore fishing. They shouted and waved as we passed by.

"On the other side of the lake there is a large cave. We think the resident dragon prevents both flooding and drying out of the lake. Everybody here believes it and we have great respect for him." Jo said as we walked along. "Tomorrow we'll go and see the Dragon Cave which stands on Dragon Hill. It's beginning to get dark so perhaps we should go back home and help prepare the special evening meal, because it's our New Year."

As soon as it grew dark a grand firework display took place in the village. Amidst the explosions of fire crackers and showers of sparkly lights from rockets, loud music erupted and people began dancing and singing on the mud-tamped paths. Everyone seemed to be happy and villagers began dropping in on Jo's family house with good wishes. They all brought little red envelopes with money in for the children. They stopped for a drink and wanted to know who I was and where I was from. I possibly caused a bit of a stir as many of these folks had never seen anything quite like me and without exception I felt welcomed. I joined the card and Mah-Jong games and smoked the local yen tong, a pipe made from a length of bamboo with tobacco in the base and water in its long tube. When you sucked hard enough through a small aperture at the top, filtered smoke came through. I'd done this on many occasions and was no novice! Eventually, amidst the loud music, drink and dancing we sat down to a delicious meal of strips of fried pork, numerous fresh vegetable cooked in the wok, noodles with chicken and big bowls of rice prepared by Jo's family. It was soon very late, and eventually, when the table was cleared, I staggered to bed feeling rather mellow and happy.

Next day we walked around the village, looking at beautiful old temples and gates which hadn't been desecrated or damaged during the Cultural Revolution of the 1970's, possibly because this hamlet was very rural and the Red Army hadn't penetrated that far. I don't know. I certainly felt very lucky to see such ancient structures.

"That's the White Dragon Cave over there," said Jo as she pointed to a dark hollow by the lake. "Can you see that tall building up there? We believe that a red dragon came one day. It annoyed the resident white dragon so much he built a very tall tower with the entrance near the top. The red dragon was very curious, and, once he got inside he was trapped and couldn't get out again. Eventually he bled to death, hence the red soil and stones that surround the site."

What a lovely story and of course, like all the villagers, I believed every word of it. My break had been a truly awe-inspiring but moving experience. This delightful family had made me really welcome. They shared what little they had and made me feel at home.

Once back in the Camellia Hotel in Kunming I began to think about work. I was about to start my final year here in China and had a lot to do. The money from the Global Issues Command was safely in Beijing. Hopefully everything would run smoothly in spite of possible communication problems. The Chinese characters totally baffled me; also, I still found it difficult to speak the language to any degree.

I reported to the foreign affairs department on my return to the Medical College before settling into my familiar flat. Nothing much had changed. The college area was still dull, grey, and unappealing, but my student friends were glad to see me and it wasn't long before I felt secure once more in my second home. The gifts I'd brought for my friends brought smiles and thanks. The two brothers, Chen Wen Jia and Chen Wen Hao, who helped me so much when I first arrived, loved their Manchester United football outfits. I don't think anyone noticed the 'Made in China' labels attached to them!

We held another successful symposium on HIV and AIDS in Lijiang, a city north of Dali. The team from the Centre for AIDS care and Research in Kunming with Dr Cheng HeHe, were a delight to work with and my interpreter was exceptional as always. Sightseeing took place in our spare time. Apart from wandering around the narrow streets and following the canals, we took a cable car to the top of Snow Mountain which towers above the city. The peak is three thousand, three hundred and fifty metres above sea level. I think if I'd known I would have requested oxygen, but off I went and fortunately had no problems. The snow-covered summit provided an extraordinary panoramic view of the neighbouring mountains and valleys. The tightly-packed city below appeared as a mass of tiled roofs, countless waterways and neatly terraced patches of vegetables and rice. The surrounding wooded areas added multiple shades of green. The experience was breath-taking.

Chapter 48

An early morning phone call from the boss disturbed my slumbers. "Peggy, Mr Martin Gordon is in town as a guest of the Security Police and, would like to meet you this evening in the Jinpeng Hotel. Be there at about five thirty tonight, and have a lovely time." And with that he was gone.

Dressed in my faithful Marks and Spencer's blue denim frock, I entered the hotel. No nerves for me this time. I was excited as memories of my London trip flooded back.

"Martin, what a lovely surprise," I exclaimed as we shook hands. "I hope you like our beautiful part of the world and that you will have time to see a little of it."

During our meal, we talked about the money that was coming our way and I told him how we planned to spend it. Looking at me, he said, "There's a head nurse at the Red Ribbon Centre in Hong Kong. Her name is Victoria Kwong and I think it would be well worth your while making a trip to see her and spending a little time in her clinic. They've been running a very successful programme for a long time. Send her an email. She may well give a presentation at the college here. She would be full of ideas."

"Wow that sounds good", I replied. "I'll certainly follow it up".

After an interesting evening I left for home, but not before agreeing to join Martin and his Security Police friends for a trip on the lake the next day.

In the morning, we boarded a small boat and cruised for couple of hours on the lake, taking in the magnificent scenery all around us. Eventually we moored in Dali town and took the local transport of horse and wagon to the legendary Butterfly Spring that lay in a valley, a short distance away. The spring water was rippling. It was clear, deep and surrounded by tall rocks. Looking at Martin I said "The local people believe that a long time ago, two lovers committed suicide to escape a cruel king. They are supposed to have jumped into the bottomless pool and became two of the hundreds of colourful butterflies that appear every May. It's a lovely story and this site is a favourite place for Chinese visitors."

Late that afternoon I left for home. I'd thoroughly enjoyed my short time with Martin and his Security Police friends, who had been surprisingly good company.

At the next meeting of the HIV and AIDS team, we talked about the grant issued from the Global Issues command. The money, ten thousand British pounds, or one hundred and thirty thousand Yuan, would be sent from the British Embassy to the VSO office in Beijing, and in turn would be allocated to us in three separate amounts. Nobody could withdraw anything without my permission, and I insisted all transactions must be written in English and Chinese, as the beautiful Chinese Characters were mostly beyond my comprehension. During the next few months we would hold workshops to train healthcare workers, teachers and prostitutes. Sadly, I couldn't persuade my colleagues to include intravenous drug abusers or the gay community at this time. They were still taboo subjects. Maybe one day somebody would listen and we would be able to get the message across to everyone. Working alongside the experts in the Dali Health Bureau, the printing and provision of HIV and AIDs educational material and the acquisition of teaching resources would take place. The existing clinic would be refurbished. We would also make the link with the condom factory, DKT in Shanghai, as requested by Simon Johnson.

The first instalment of the donation arrived almost immediately. I felt a huge responsibility land on my shoulders; it was a lot of money. But my fears were laid to rest when I sat down with the team and my boss, who I hadn't always trusted. He had changed and offered his full support. Estimates had been received for the upgrade of the clinic, and we decided to use a local company to carry out the work. Professor Yang Ting Shi from the Public Health Department had expressed a growing concern for the spread of HIV and AIDS within the Prefecture and wanted to get his research project on local knowledge, attitudes and beliefs underway. It was therefore with complete confidence that I signed the first cheques and felt good as my colleagues co-signed them. I faxed copies of the agreements and cheques to both VSO and Simon at the Embassy to keep them in the loop.

Dates were planned to give weekend training courses to as many persons as possible that might be in contact with HIV and AIDS. My colleagues sought permission and approval from relative health officials, and we were able to print thousands of information leaflets and booklets to give all course participants at least one copy. All was going well apart from linking up with the condom factory in Shanghai. I'd never know the reason for this reluctance and guessed that someone, somewhere, in the hierarchy, didn't support the use of this essential item. I found this hard to accept, because I was used to condoms being readily available in many outlets at home. But I was in China and had to obey the college 'experts' and go along with it.

In Hong Kong, Victoria Kwong was delighted to receive my e-mail. She suggested giving a three-day session at the Medical College at the end of the May. She would bring posters and medical teaching books regarding STDs and HIV and AIDS, and looked forward to visiting us. I talked to my boss as we made arrangements for her visit. He actually agreed that her experience would be invaluable, and wanted to meet her. Although Cantonese was the principle language spoken in Hong Kong, all the books would be printed in Chinese Characters, which was fine.

When Victoria arrived, we sat and chatted. She was a petite little soul with a beautiful smile. "I'm really glad you asked me to come. I've never been here before and I hope we'll have time to look around; it looks and feels gorgeous. So much space, and that's something we don't have where I come from."

she said, as she laughed. "And, with regards to my lectures, I'm going to tell them what we do in our clinic, like educating the general public, and offering support and training to all those involved with the virus. We also work with many others, both locally and internationally. Since we opened in 1997, literally hundreds of people have passed through our doors. We never turn anyone away, irrespective of colour, creed or sexuality. At some stage, I will discuss the virus and latest treatments and I understand you are going to tell them how the disease is spread and the care patients and their families will need. This should be a good couple of days."

I liked this girl a lot. She was easy to get on with and was obviously very able.

During her sessions, literally hundreds of doctors and nurses came to listen to and learn. I was delighted to listen to her lectures, which included information for the gay community on the use of condoms for all sexual activity and how intravenous drug users were encouraged to use new needles and syringes each time they needed a top up.

And, from our pot of money, we were able to cover all expenses. It felt good and I thought we were really getting somewhere at last. As she was leaving, Victoria gave me two text books, the EU book on Sexually Transmitted Diseases, which she had brought. I gave one to the doctors who had created the clinic. The other I decided to give to Jianbuo, at the Number Two People's Hospital in Dali, because I knew how seriously he took his work. She rewarded me with an invitation to Hong Kong, which I readily accepted. That afternoon I spent time with my boss discussing the success of Victoria's visit and told him about my invitation to spend a few days with her.

"Go," he said. "You will learn a lot. It will be good experience and I support you all the way. And, while you've been occupied this week the clinic has been fixed. Go and have a look. You'll have a big surprise."

I took a taxi and could hardly believe my eyes. The place had been totally refurbished and the change was dramatic. The whole unit had been repaired and repainted with a brilliant white paint. Running water had been connected to a new hand washbasin in the treatment room on the ground floor. On the first floor, bright curtains had been erected around the examination couches and matching sheets and duvets covered the beds in the 'women's' department. I couldn't imagine having a check-up without privacy, but I'd long since learned about expectations and guessed, if there was no curtain, that's the way it had to be. I wondered what the clients thought about the changes. On the second floor, a counselling room had been created and was well-appointed with a small table, a huge flask and a couple of mugs, and two easy chairs, with bright flowery curtains hanging at the windows. On the flat roof, an electric shower unit had been installed in a small room. It was within easy reach and simple to use. I spent time with the health professionals who were overjoyed at the improvements to their clinic.

The next few weeks were hectic, planning weekend training sessions for our own health care workers, teachers and their senior students, and prostitutes. Although a lot of these individuals had been to our training sessions in the past, there were hundreds more who needed help and advice. It was almost like starting from scratch, and the first group to arrive at the college was a noisy set of sixty or so barefoot doctors. Most of these folks had received as little as six weeks medical training, but had acquired a lot of knowledge as they went about their daily work. Their roles were invaluable in remote rural communities. Accommodation and food was provided by the college, and it was a sheer pleasure to fund this group of mainly poor village farmers, who were keen and wanted to know so much. Over the next few months we spread awareness to the many individuals who might come in contact with the then dreaded disease. It was decided that our own doctors would visit nightclubs, brothels and bordellos where prostitutes practised what they did best. They would encourage these girls to spread the word to as many of their co-workers as possible. Some of these girls were only fifteen or sixteen, or even younger. My original interpreter, Rumei, and I were invited to several women's groups. During and after our presentations on HIV and AIDS, we were bombarded with questions from these ordinary people, the wives and mothers who would be the carers if their husbands or offspring became infected with the virus. They particularly loved my use of a banana to show them how a condom should be applied. It caused an absolute uproar as most had never seen a condom, let alone touched one. I felt relaxed in their company and it seemed they felt the same, too.

It was end of June when an excited me boarded the night bus to Kunming on my way to Hong Kong. This was more new ground for me. I'd always wanted to visit this interesting capitalistic island standing on the very edge of Communist China. In addition, I wanted to see Victoria again. She had recommended the YMCA in Kowloon for my stay, as it was fairly close to her place of work. I felt a little anxious about this, but needn't have worried because I was given a good clean room with bathroom on a floor reserved for females only. I slept well that night.

Feeling rested after a good night's sleep, I found her clinic and ventured through the doors of her office. "Welcome," she said, "You've only got a few days here, so I'll show you round the clinic first. Please feel free to ask me, or any of my staff questions, and we'll do our best to answer them. I wish you all the luck in the world with your task, but remember it takes time and patience. We've been operating for two years now, and in that time, we've all learned so much. Get some sight-seeing in and come back before you leave as I've got some 'stuff' for you. And I hope you've got an empty bag!" With her words ringing in my ears I left.

What 'stuff' was I going to get? I wondered, but knew I'd soon find out! I spent that day, and the next, alternating my time between the clinic and exploring the surrounding area. I'd met a pretty Irish girl called Anne at the YMCA. She'd come for a job interview, and we hit it off immediately. Together we walked around the brightly lit shops and market stalls, finding them crammed with assorted interesting items. We couldn't resist buying colourful cotton tops and a couple of pairs of blue jeans. We rested at a roadside café, ate delicious cakes and washed them down with iced Cokes. Later we visited Kowloon Park and the Kowloon Mosque which stood nearby. We'd enjoyed our bit of sight-seeing and I felt sad at having to return to China so soon.

Late afternoon on the day of my departure I went to the clinic to collect my 'stuff'. Victoria was laughing as I gazed at the pile of textbooks concerning STD's, the large collection of multi-coloured Durex condoms and a couple of artificial penises made of a soft rubbery substance. They had been painted and looked almost real!

She explained "I thought this gear would be more than useful to you, especially when you are showing people how to use condoms, but I'm sure you know that already".

We laughed as I told her I used a banana for demonstrations. "There are loads of bananas, but my supply of condoms is fast running out, and they don't appear to be readily available in my part of the world. I'm chuffed with your gifts and pray that I don't have to go through a search at either of the airports. Bye, Victoria, and thank you so much." I managed to cram all the goodies into my bag, and set off for home.

My return journey was uneventful. No searches for me at either airport, to my utter relief, and I quickly settled back into my routine with my goodies kept hidden in my flat! I went to see Jianbuo at Dali No. Two Peoples Hospital and gave him an assortment of Durex condoms to help him teach the local prostitutes the value of these items. I also went to my friend in the café and gave him a collection which he would keep 'under the counter' to give to his friends, should the need arise! Why did these items have to be so secret, I wondered? After all it was 1999!

We were due another weekend training session, and I would be able to officially familiarise one of my new penile forms and jazzy condoms to a group of doctors from the rural areas. I couldn't think of a better group for this introduction, and indeed it worked. The men were shy and hid their faces in embarrassment, but the ladies came to the fore and could hardly believe their eyes when I tipped the box of assorted colours and shapes of the Durex condoms. They all laughed when I said one of our English slang words for then was 'johnnies'. They fitted them onto the artificial penises with no problem, and smiled proudly as they showed the audience their new-found skill. Happy days – I was getting there at last, well almost.

At our final team meeting before the summer break, the squad promised to continue the work. With the agreement of everyone it was decided the outreach clinic staff would receive more training, and the public health team would organise some senior medical students to carry out a survey about HIV and AIDS in their home towns or villages before we embarked on a much larger awareness programme throughout the prefecture.

The first two instalments of our grant had been used, and after I'd checked the receipts, the third and final payment was requested. This amazing donation from the British Government had made a huge difference to me and the team in our efforts to make so many ordinary people aware of the HIV problem; it also seemed to spur the political hierarchy into action and I was thrilled to bits. Hopefully we would be able to reach many people, not only health workers, but ordinary members of society in the Dali area and provide an awareness of the situation, allowing them to take the necessary precautions and care for themselves. I had grown to love many of these people and didn't want to think of any of them dying through ignorance. It was immaterial to me should they be prostitutes, intravenous drug users, gays, or babies who had been infected by their mothers; they were people like me and deserved a reasonable quality of life, however poor they may have been and it seemed all the team members were feeling the same.

That evening I sat and thought about Dr Prakong and her husband in Thailand. They had both worked tirelessly for years to achieve the present HIV and AIDS awareness level in Chiang Mai. Here, in this corner of China, we were starting a new adventure and I knew there was a long, long way to go.

I emailed the latest news and a report to VSO and Simon at the Embassy. But now I was off to the 'land of smiles' for a holiday, and after securing my visas, headed off to Kunming to catch my flight to Chiang Mai.

Chapter 49

Because I worked in a medical college, my holidays were always that bit longer than my VSO teacher colleagues. I didn't mind, and was happy to link up with old friends in Chiang Mai or unwind on my own for a week or two. I knew about the terrible tragedy that had occurred in Cambodia in the seventies, and decided to spend a few days in Phnom Penh and surrounding area. On a visit to a travel shop in the city, the agent said, "Yes, you can go to Cambodia, but it's not wise to go alone. I will arrange a government guide to meet you at the Airport. It won't cost you too much. If you haven't found a hotel, may I suggest the Sheratton? It's central and safe." I accepted his advice and booked the short flight for the next day.

On arrival in Phnom Penh I could see a man holding a placard displaying my name. He was aged about 30, smartly dressed, slim, of small stature and had Chinese features. His face lit up as I approached him and said "hello".

"Hi, my name's Chakara and I'll be looking after you during your time here. Welcome to Cambodia," he said, making me feel at ease. "I'll take you to your hotel, let you unpack and later on we'll go out for a meal."

I replied, "OK, let's go," and we went in his car to the hotel.

It may well have been called the Sheratton, but it was nothing like a hotel of similar name I'd used in the UK. Perhaps that's why the spelling was different, and why the facilities were poor to say the least. But I had a shower unit in my room, the bed was clean and there was a good lock on the door, so I felt reasonably content.

As we drove the short distance to a restaurant, I could see shell-damaged old French style houses and shops. Bullet holes, clearly visible on many properties, spoke for themselves. My guide shook his head, "There was a lot of devastation during the three-year struggle we endured with our infamous leader Pol Pot and his Khmer Rouge Army. It was sheer hell from 1975 to 1978. I'll tell you more as we go along".

With that he parked his four-wheel drive on the roadside in front of a restaurant, and gave some money to a young man. I watched the financial transaction take place and wondered what it was all about, until a scooter sped by. The young rider and his mate on the back both had revolvers poking out from their jeans' pockets. "These young men will steal anything, including my car, and believe me they're not afraid to use their guns," I was told, and quite suddenly I was relieved to have my own personal protector.

As we entered the dimly lit cafe I could see smoke rising above a wire-topped brazier standing over charcoal-filled clay pots at the back of the room. Walking towards the smoke, I could see rows and rows of sizzling small fish. They looked good, and I wished I could smell them, but, even so, I thoroughly enjoyed my meal of fish, sliced cucumber and tomatoes, all topped with a garlic sauce and lime juice. A couple of glasses of dry white wine enhanced the fantastic sweet and sour flavour, and my guide and I spent an interesting hour or two getting to know each other.

The following morning over a breakfast of strong black coffee and crispy rolls (the French influence was still alive and well) Chakara suggested how my four-day visit would be best spent. "Today I'll take you to the Tuol Sleng Museum and tomorrow we'll go to the Killing Fields. That leaves the Angkor Wat for you to see and enjoy before you return to Thailand. How does that sound? I've left Angkor Wat until last, because I think you'll need a break by then. We'll have to find accommodation for you there as well, because we'll stay overnight."

I replied, "Sounds fine to me. I'm depending on you to guide me, because it's your country and you know the most interesting places for visitors to see."

We stood in the playground of the former Chao Ponhea Yat High School. The shadows of the tall, graceful palm trees that lined the schoolyard gave little or no respite from the scorching heat. These same shadows gave no clue to the horror that was to confront me as we entered the museum, one of five buildings within the complex.

On walking through the entrance, I was confronted with wall after wall of disturbing photographs of men, women and children. They were all named, numbered and dated by boards

321

on their chests. Any preparation I had made mentally for this visit evaporated, and I felt sickened by the sight of the frightened faces that stared back at me. Chakara looked down and took a deep breath, "The Khmer Rouge Leaders kept a meticulous record of their brutality. As you can see many of these people were photographed before and after torture, and altogether some seventeen thousand people, mainly Cambodians died either here, or in the Killing Fields, a short distance away. And that's only in Phnom Penh. There were many children and babies, too. All murdered and only seven people survived."

He walked away with tears in his eyes, leaving me to wander silently around the area, and gaze at the endless rows of faces, trying desperately to fathom out the reason for this dreadful atrocity.

"Some of my relatives died here," my guide whispered and pointed to a grainy photo. "This was my uncle and the only crime he committed was to wear glasses. The Khmer Rouge Leaders were crazy, and even some of their executioners and torturers were routinely killed and replaced by others desperate to take their positions. We were liberated eventually by the Vietnamese Army in 1978, and are still trying to come to terms with this barbaric act of insanity."

I took a long, deep breath and tried to compose myself as we toured the rest of the museum. In former classrooms, I saw rusty iron beds with leg shackles still attached "The liberating soldiers took photographs of the dead as they found them, and these large pictures hanging on the walls are the remains of victims, still on their beds" said my guide. "Come with me," said Chakara. "This room is full of tiny brick cells the hostages had to build. No water and no ventilation."

I looked in at the cells, complete with leg shackles, and felt there was barely room to stand. I tried to imagine how it must have been for the poor souls who were forced to sit in complete silence for hours on end. I couldn't. In the next room hundreds of victims were chained to a central bar. "They couldn't move and if they made any noise they were severely beaten by guards, some as young as twelve or thirteen." My guide said.

Our final visit that day was to a special room dedicated to one of the few survivors. "Vann Nath is an accomplished artist, and these terrible scenes were painted as he witnessed them. He probably survived because of his expertise, and it was done firstly to record what actually happened, and secondly to help him recover from his ordeal. He still paints today said Chakara quietly.

I studied the graphic paintings, one by one. A man, tied by his legs, was lying on the floor receiving lashes by four men holding whips. Another, with his hands and legs shackled, was being given electric shocks to his chest. A young woman, trying in vain to hold on to her baby as it was forcibly taken from her by a young man in some sort of uniform. A man wielding a bayonet was aiming at another baby as it was thrown high into the air by another man. The explicit scenes of dead or dying people in such grotesque positions made me feel ill and I turned away with tears running down my face.

My guide took my arm and said in a low voice, "These poor people were fed only watery gruel once a day and were hosed down every four days. Do you want to go now? I think you've seen enough." he asked.

"Yes, please Chakara," I gulped, and we left the building.

That evening I wept as I updated my diary. My day had been a profoundly sad experience, and I'd gained a true picture of man's inhumanity to man. I didn't sleep well that night.

Next morning, we set off for the Killing Fields at Choeung Ek, a few miles out of Phnom Penh. This area was one of hundreds of other such sites around Cambodia, where the Khmer Rouge practiced their genocide. On the way, we stopped at a roadside café and drank strong black coffee, partly because I felt this might give me the courage to face more horrifying scenes. As we parked at Choeung Ek, the place looked almost deserted, apart from a few tourists milling about. Looking straight ahead, I was confronted with the sight of the now famous glass shrine, full of human skulls. I'd felt wretched when I'd had a glimpse of this a few years ago on UK television, but now I was faced with the real thing I felt even more depressed.

"There are eight thousand skulls stored in there," Chakara said "and, maybe what's even worse, these uneven fields contain mass graves for perhaps twenty thousand Cambodians. We'll never know."

I stood still and wondered how Chakara felt. These were his people, his family even, lying under our feet, and yet he was comforting me, a complete outsider. It must have been difficult for him.

"There's more to see over there,"

As we walked along a tree lined avenue, beneath our feet, the mud-tamped path revealed scraps of cloth, human teeth and shards of bone. "Nooses were hung from these trees. This was one of the hanging zones." I looked up and could see frayed remnants of ropes above me. I couldn't speak and remained silent till we reached to a large tree, the bark of which was scarred and dented. "Do you remember that painting of blind-folded little boys holding hands in the Tuol Sleng museum? This is where some of them met their end. They were grasped by the legs and beaten against this lovely old tree until they were dead."

At this point I'd had enough. "Please, take me back to Phnom Penh" I said. "I've seen more than enough", and with that we left.

Back in the war-scarred city, Chakara took me to a beautiful Buddhist Temple, where, with a glass of green tea, I sat alone and reflected. The mind-blowing experiences, I had voluntarily undergone affected me deeply; I felt sickened and numb. After a while, I realised I had to accept the fact that this slaughter of innocents had occurred, and it was time for me to move on. I would never forget the scenes I'd witnessed, or the stories my guide told me, and to this day I still weep at the memory of it all. I will never understand how man can be so cruel.

We made an early start to see the famous Temple, or Wat, at Angkor in Cambodia's most Northern Province of Siem Reap. After a long hot journey in a tatty old bus the Temple was an absolute joy to see, and nothing like the images I had previously been shown. The size and scale was overwhelming and I knew this was something great and spiritual. In a little café, near the entrance, Chakara began to give me a few facts.

"This wonderful temple was first built during the 12th century. It was originally a Hindu Shrine representing the universe, and dedicated to the god Vishnu. In the 13th century it became a Buddhist Temple; it's the world's largest religious structure and has never been abandoned. As you can see it's used today. It gives peace and happiness to us Cambodians, and as a nation we are very proud of it. It occupies a huge space and contains many small sanctuaries, the main one being Mount Meru, representing the home of the ancient gods. Although the Khmer Army did some damage during Pol Pot's time, it's slowly but surely being repaired." I looked up and saw a myriad of red sandstone towers, dozens of sets of steps leading upwards and a few orange clad monks milling around.

We crossed the wide moat surrounding the temple and I was totally blown away by the enormity of the place. As we drew nearer the entrance I could see the outer walls were beautifully decorated with carvings of celestial dancers.

"These dancers surround the whole building and each one is different. Let's go inside, where you'll see hundreds of carvings portraying historical events and stories from mythology," said Chakara.

We spent the next three or four hours wandering up the stairways, studying intricate carvings, looking inside small shrines, and paying respects to the Buddhas in many temples. In places, large vines flourished between the sandstone buildings, adding more mystery to this sacred place. Sometimes nature can be more spiritually dramatic than anything man can create.

Chakara smiled and said "We will go to Siem Reap now to find you a hotel room and come back here in the morning at sunrise. I know you will love it."

Early next morning we arrived at Angkor Wat just as an orange sun was rising over the sandstone towers. Chakara and I stood in silence by the moat as shadows and reflections danced all around. I felt calm and totally at peace, a much-needed break after my recent experiences. To me, this example of ancient Khmer architecture was so much more than a temple; it was a spiritual haven and I was at a loss for words.

Before my short time in Cambodia came to an end, I thanked Chakara, not only for his choice of visits, but also his care and thoughtful approach towards me. He started out as a government guide, but ended up being my friend. I couldn't do much, but handed him my wristwatch as a 'thank you' gift because I knew he didn't have one. He was the great guy who made my trip so memorable.

Back in Thailand I met three VSO teacher friends and we spent the next month hopping between Koh Samui and Koh Phi Phi, two small islands off the southern Thai coast. We swam, we drank, and we ate well and slept on the sands in thatched huts with basic facilities. With bleached-white beaches and surrounding jungles the islands were idyllic, the only disturbance being the put-put of the long-boat engines as boatmen cruised around the odd craggy rock that went down to the sea. A little bit of heaven on earth.

Before I returned to China I called to see Dr Prakong at Chiang Mai University to let her know of my progress with the HIV problem in Dali. She was delighted with my news and promised once more to help in any way she could. She shared my disappointment with the lack of any contact from the medical college in Dali regarding post graduate training for doctors on HIV and AIDS. Maybe, one day, but thoughts in China were so different from those in Thailand.

All too soon the holiday was over. I'd had a memorable experience in Cambodia followed by a fantastic break with my VSO colleagues, and we looked forward to meeting up again at the annual VSO Conference in November, but right now it was back to China.

Chapter 50

But now it was September and I was entering the final phase of my placement at Dali Medical College in the beautiful Province of Yunnan in The Peoples Republic of China.

My first port of call was as ever to the post room to collect mail from home; always a happy time for me and I was never disappointed, thank heaven for family and friends. Next, I checked in with my boss who greeted me with a huge smile. "I hope you've had a good holiday and I'm glad you're back. Before I forget, there's a message for you from VSO. A doctor named William Wong has taken a placement in the medical department of Kunming University. Give him a ring and perhaps meet up with him. Now, back to work, you'll be pleased to hear that we've contacted DKT, the condom company in Shanghai. The representative has paid us a visit, left a mountain of samples, and will be more than happy to attend your next teaching sessions. When you have time, go down to the new clinic and take some of these samples together with two or three of those posters you brought back from Hong Kong. The doctors and nurses will be pleased to see you. A meeting has been arranged for your team on Monday morning, and I'll see you then."

I had to smile, remembering eighteen months ago when I informed him that his doctors wanted to know about HIV and AIDS. With anger in his face he had bellowed, "There's no problem here in China. It's you, in the decadent West who is to blame." Now, here he was, sitting with a big grin on his face, planning my last few weeks at his college. I was very glad he had changed his views.

The next day I went to the clinic where I handed over the box of condoms. With the huge population, I secretly wondered how long one hundred would last, but hoped, if nothing else, it would at least introduce people to the concept of contraception and prevent many sexually transmitted diseases. Time would tell, and I guessed the medics would have a lot of educating to do with the prostitutes and rent boys, because Chinese men would be no different to rest the of the world's male population in their dislike of these items! The nurses loved the posters with their Chinese character comments; they giggled as they studied the colourful comical drawings portraying the value of a condom for any sexual activity at all times. They wasted no time in sticking them on the pristine walls for all to see. A successful mission!

That evening I contacted William in Kunming and arranged to meet him the following weekend. I booked a bed on the sleeper bus and a room in my favourite hotel, the Camellia in Kunming, taking advantage of the special rates now given to me and travelled to Kunming on the Friday evening.

Grabbing a taxi to the university I found William waiting at the gated entrance. Over coffee and a snack we chatted non-stop. He was Chinese, but had lived in the United Kingdom for much of his life and had graduated in medicine. He had decided to spend time in China, was bilingual and had taken up a post at the university with VSO. I met his wife, Skye and their two little girls. They lived in a flat, not dissimilar to mine, within the university complex,

That weekend I became his tour guide and when I left for home on the Sunday evening we promised to keep in touch. Over the next weekends he visited me at the Medical College taking advantage of the guest rooms available. He updated me on the many advances made in the worldwide fight against HIV and AIDS and how I wished he had been around during my early days. Over the next few months we met frequently and I was able to introduce him to my NGO friends in the city.

During one of these weekends I took William to Dali and over a meal in Jack's Café introduced him to Jianbuo. After a while I sat and chatted to Jack while these two young doctors put their heads together. They seemed to get on well, both speaking the same language. I knew William would advise Jianbuo on the many aspects of HIV which was of interest to both of them. It wasn't long before they became good friends and would keep in touch.

Monday arrived and as I walked into the meeting room, my colleagues smiled and welcomed me. The monetary donation had made a huge difference in this poverty-stricken area, and, with the help it provided, everyone was motivated and keen to continue efforts to alert and educate the local population to the dangers of HIV.

"A lot has happened in the out-reach clinic," said Francis. "The health professionals who work there now know about the special needs of those who come with a sexually transmitted disease, and the risk of an HIV infection. They have had training in counselling as well and the doctor in charge of the clinic is so pleased with the results. Jimmy and I are delighted."

Professor Yang Ting Shi spoke next. "As you know Yunnan is a very poor Province, and there isn't the money to spend on educational material. During the summer holidays, some of our senior medical students carried out week-long campaigns in their home towns or villages and have come up with interesting results. Over two thousand members of the general public attended. Most of them had heard about HIV, but didn't know how it was spread. They knew it was a serious disease and were afraid of it. A quarter of those interviewed felt anyone with HIV or AIDS deserved it because they were either junkies or prostitutes."

As I listened I wondered why there had been no mention of the gay community, or a needle and syringe exchange policy, but no doubt I was hoping for too much.

Before the meeting ended, one more teaching session was arranged for our nurses and doctors, also an educational and awareness operation throughout the Prefecture was organised. It would take the shape of a publicity campaign in each of the fifteen major towns and it would be a research project looking into the knowledge, attitudes and thoughts of the general public regarding HIV and AIDS. Questionnaires were designed, and after approval by the local health bureau, thousands were printed together with the information leaflets. I was going to be busy in my last few weeks in China, with the county awareness campaign, a study weekend at the college, the annual VSO conference in Xi'an, and World AIDS Day on the 1st December, in which I would again take an active role.

Inside the main office in the Public Health Department, it looked as if a gang of school kids had dumped their 'stuff' and left in a hurry. On one table sat a stack of the EU textbooks on Sexually Transmitted Diseases which I had requested from VSO, and next to them sat my enlarged photographs of some of the Thai children, who had been infected with HIV by their pregnant mothers. There were also paintings, posters, condoms, information leaflets, six large sheets of plywood, a couple of rolls of white plastic sheeting, five long Bungee cords and a large roll of twine shoved into corners and piled on tables.

"Hi Peggy," said the Professor from behind a sheet of plywood. "We are preparing the visual aids for our publicity campaign and you've come just in time. We've got four days to get everything ready, and once we've sorted out these bill-boards, we can discuss our plans for the meetings which will call roadshows. They must be simple, informative and interesting. I'm looking forward to the final results of the survey."

I trusted this pleasant man implicitly. He was wise and very experienced, knowing exactly how to get this important message across to his own people, whose cultures were so different to mine. Now he had the opportunity, just as Rumei my previous interpreter had done before, and I knew he would do well. I had a particularly good relationship with his group of public health experts. We laughed and chatted as we glued the artworks on to the large pieces of plywood, before wrapping them in white plastic sheets. They were all different and eye-catching. We stockpiled thousands of information leaflets, and as many condoms as we could lay our hands on, in readiness for our task which would start the following weekend. For me, this venture offered not only a wonderful opportunity to travel and meet new people, but also provide an insight into the lives of ordinary folk in some of the more remote areas which I had only been able to read about in my Lonely Planet guide book. I was curious and excited.

The day of our first campaign arrived. At sunrise, the six of us made our way to the bus station, a fifteen-minute walk away. No college transport this time, it was pick up your stuff and walk! We must have looked an odd sight carrying an assortment of bags and bill-boards covered in white plastic sheeting and tied up with twine, but perhaps not, as anything seemed to be acceptable in this country. The doctor had informed us that having had breakfast at the bus station, we should buy water as the journey would take at least three hours. Other destinations would take a lot longer.

With our bill-boards secured on the roof of the crowded mini-bus, we set off. On this occasion, we were accompanied by two goats roped to a rear seat, a number of squealing piglets tied in a hessian sack, numerous chickens with their legs tied together sitting silently on the axle housing, and a bucket full of live fish next to the driver. This was not unusual and became the norm for most of our trips in this beautiful rural area. With the constant lighting of cigarettes and the hawking, coughing and spitting, together with the smells of the animals, the air must have been like farmyard smog by the time we reached our destination. I was truly grateful to be totally unaware of the stench, but that was travelling in rural china and I was well used to it!

On arrival at the selected areas, we had to locate the Party Secretary and a local government official to gain permission to set up our roadshow in the town or village square. The day chosen should be the local market day where most of the population would be attending.

During the next eight weeks, we visited twelve county towns, most of which consisted of rows of gloomy-looking mud-walled single-storey dwellings which lined the roads and lanes. As normal in this part of the world, multiple electric cables trailed from lamp posts to corners of buildings and dangled dangerously close to our heads, or so it seemed. I doubted that the party members, government officials and medical teams who supported and welcomed us so warmly, lived in those tiny homes. I'd never know.

From the anti-epidemic teams and local doctors, who worked in the General Hospitals and Traditional Chinese Hospitals, I learned about the increasing numbers of people attending clinics with STDs and tuberculosis in one form or another. Not one of the towns we visited had any blood testing facilities, so diagnosis was difficult and expensive. Medical treatment was not free and many people were so poor they couldn't afford even the simplest care so often didn't seek it. Thus no proper records could be kept. There was little employment in any of the towns we visited, where most adults scratched some sort of a living from agriculture. I felt sorry for the medics. They were doing their best and were more than happy to take any teaching aids we were able to give them. A senior doctor in each town was presented with a copy of the EU book on STDs. They were grateful and promised to share the information with their colleagues. There were few, if any, newspapers available, and most of the towns used a blackboard and chalk system to spread information. Everyday someone would update the blackboard which stood in a prominent position in the square and crowds would gather round to read the latest news bulletin.

Our roadshows caused a great deal of interest, and hundreds of people of all ages crowded around us in each town we visited. They read the information leaflets, examined the condoms and listened intently as our doctors told them of the dangers of unprotected sex, also the sharing of needles and syringes within the drug taking communities. They explained how the HIV infection, and others diseases like Hepatitis B, was passed from person to person through infected blood, and told them of ways they could protect themselves. Few asked questions, but our team of experts kept repeating the three ways the virus could be spread from person to person, and tried to make sure each one understood, in language which these poorly educated people could comprehend.

Local television was always present, and I became a celebrity of some sort because many people had never seen anything like me before. I was a foreigner, or foreign devil *'guizi,'* as they sometimes called me. I had my arms felt, my brown hair stroked and my blue eyes stared into. I smiled at these folk, who were, by nature, inquisitive and suspicious, and continued pushing information leaflets into their small, dirty brown hands. Sometimes I moved away from the market squares into the surrounding districts where I found shop keepers, builders, and farmers, all keen to know what was going on. They were more than happy to receive the information on HIV. During these visits, I also met many people from different ethnic minority groups including Hui, Yi, Miao, Bai, Buran, Lisu, Naxi, Hani, Dai, Lahu, Wa, Zhang and Yao. Most of the women wore their distinctive, colourful costumes which had been retained for generations. They were proud people. Their features were different from many of the Han Chinese I knew, and they spoke in their own dialects which made conversation with me impossible, but it was amazing what their eyes said and I always felt comfortable in their company. Occasionally they would gather their children and demand a photo. I was more than happy to oblige, because I love all children. I was more than fortunate to have the Professor to translate for me when he had a few minutes to spare. These were intimate and happy times for me.

Some of the remote towns we visited were in the north of the county and were rarely, if ever, visited by foreigners. During these times, I was given a personal security guard to watch over me and keep me safe, or was it to stop me seeing certain bodily activities like urinating, or worse, in doorways or by the roadside. I never did find out, but I had been here long enough to know that this happened, and I'd just look the other way. This skinny little man, whose name was Dong, wore a green suit at least two sizes too big for him. He was pleasant enough though, and enjoyed the cigarettes and beers I bought him. The poor soul had to sleep on a hard chair outside my hotel room, to check I didn't wander off?? And thinking of hotels, why, oh why, are hotels for foreigners in some places so disgustingly filthy? The carpets were threadbare, covered in cigarette burns and had suspicious looking dark stains which might, or might not have been, spilt coffee. Bathrooms were grubby, and toilets often wouldn't flush unless assisted by a couple of waste-paper bins of water filched from the tap in the hand wash-basin. The single beds were fine, with freshly laundered sheets and pillow slips, but I still used my own small towel to cover the pillow. I never investigated further, frightened of what I might find, knowing I had to accept what was offered. Sharing accommodation with my colleagues was taboo, as theirs was for Chinese only. As I'd had a personal experience in Lijiang with Toshi, the Japanese guy, and Wu Ling, the teacher from Dali, a while ago, I didn't even ask about their conditions. With my door firmly bolted, I managed to sleep well each night, in spite of the general griminess. I shared all meals with my colleagues, but Dong wasn't allowed to join us. He would disappear around the back of whichever friendly, smoke-blackened little eating place we chose, and re-appear as soon as we were ready to go. He trotted faithfully along behind me everywhere we went, confiscating my camera whenever he felt it necessary, like on the occasion I was allowed into a drug rehabilitation centre to meet and talk to inmates with an interpreter. The six young men I met looked miserable and fed up, which I could understand. They chatted to my interpreter as they showed me their sleeping area which contained bed-rolls on a wooden floor. A small pile of plastic eating tools and mugs sat next to the bundles. Apart from that room, which contained a concrete shelf with a tap fitted above it, a hut which contained a squat toilet and a well-kept yard for exercise, it seemed they had little else.

My interpreter told me, "This unit has a poor success rate, as most of the inmates' families find money from somewhere and make secret deliveries, so the drug use continues. I think it's possibly because people don't understand what rehabilitation is all about. It's a sad situation, and I doubt if this place is unique. The men and women employed here do what they can while these addicts are resident, but when they go, well, it's anybody's guess."

With twelve county towns visited, we had to take a break and return to the college, where I went to see my boss. After the usual greeting, he said, "Peggy, I've been told you've all done well and achieved your aims in all the towns you've been to. Unfortunately, I'm not in a position to grant you permission to visit the last three towns which are in the north of the county. I'm sorry, but that's it."

Receiving no explanation whatsoever, I was shown out of his office. Standing in the corridor I felt devastated and needed to talk to someone and decided to see Professor Yang Ting Shi. This project had been close to his heart and I knew he'd be upset. He'd already received the news when I met him and was as upset as I was.

"I understood there was enough time and grant money to complete the survey and that was part of the deal," he grumbled

I said, "But there's nothing I can do. David has said no, and he means it. Perhaps it's something to do with the extreme poverty, suffering, and lack of care that I've seen in some places? I don't know. But what I do know is that you and your team won't be able to complete the survey, unless perhaps, when I've gone back to England you will be allowed to continue. I do hope so," I said.

The Professor, with sadness in his voice replied, "I'm sorry too, but all isn't lost because think of the hundreds and hundreds of people of all ages we've been able to talk to and give simple information and advice. The television coverage has been extraordinary as well, and the companies will repeat their programmes time and time again to reach a much wider audience. My colleagues and I spoke to the crowds in a language they all understood, translating for you when you told them about condoms and the hazards of any unprotected sex. Also, how babies could be infected if their mothers suffered from HIV during pregnancy. We encouraged the use of latex gloves by doctors and nurses to minimise the risks with contaminated blood, not only from infected patients in hospitals and clinics, but also from intravenous drug users who may carry HIV, or other blood-borne diseases. Everyone needs to be careful, but even more so where there are no blood testing facilities. You, the foreign devil, or *'guizi,'* as they originally thought of you, were the centre of attention and they will remember both you and the message you brought for a long time to come. You walked amongst them and they made you welcome, that's a deal in itself. You did well and were good company and we enjoyed having you with us."

I smiled and said, "I've learned such a lot about the lives of ordinary folk in these isolated places and I want to say how well you not only looked after me on my journey into the unknown, but also kept me informed throughout. You've got a wonderful Public Health team, Professor, thank you so very much for all you've done, and tonight we're all going out for a celebratory meal on me."

That evening we had a feast of noodles and thin strips of chicken, sweet and sour pork in batter, small spicy pork filled steamed buns, shreds of boiled cabbage floating in water, rice, tender bamboo shoots, pickled cabbage and gherkins, and of course the obligatory hot, hot chilli sauce, all washed down with a number of Dali beers. We were a happy bunch of like-minded people who had achieved an ambition of spreading awareness of HIV in many parts of the county, and we celebrated in style!

The next week brought the promised two-day session for forty senior doctors and nurses. These people had attended our courses in the past, and had been invited to tell us about their personal achievements in teaching their colleagues, families and friends about the dangers of HIV and other blood-borne diseases. I listened intently as my interpreter translated the presentations, and I was impressed. They'd touched on all the aspects they had been taught, especially the hazards of infected blood and unprotected sex, and I thought back to the days when Rumei interpreted my lectures during our teaching sessions in the past. She, like the Professor and his team, had certainly known how to get the message across to their own people and do it in such a way that they could all get to grips with the situation. For the first time at the college a representative from the DKT condom company in Shanghai was present with leaflets and samples for all present. He was given a stand in a prominent position, and had a busy couple of days chatting to the doctors and nurses in a relaxed and friendly atmosphere. It was rewarding to see, and I realised how times had changed in such a short while. I was delighted. On the final day my friend Jianbuo gave a moving account of his personal care and treatment to the two young AIDS patients in the No. two Hospital in Dali. The woman, a teenage prostitute, had become infected, possibly through unprotected sex, and the young man had used intravenous drugs, sharing needles and syringes with his friends. Both had died through ignorance and the doctor had cared for both his patients and their families. He certainly deserved the standing ovation, and the credit he received at the end of his presentation. The previous week this same doctor had the first article ever on HIV and AIDS published in the local paper. That was good news for the resident population and I applauded him for his efforts. The doctor and I had been friends for a long time, and although he could speak little or no English, I always knew this man was something special.

The following week I went to Xi'an for my final VSO Conference. This annual three-day event drew the volunteers together from all over China, a time when we could all relax and enjoy each other's company. For me it was a bitter sweet affair, meeting new people whilst saying goodbye to those I had known for a short while, both volunteers and programme officers. All the people I'd originally travelled out with three years ago had returned to the United Kingdom, but there were others I'd met the previous year, and we hoped we might meet again at one of the VSO de-briefing weekends in Birmingham.

I returned to Xiaguan, knowing it was my turn to be repatriated in a few weeks, and I felt good.

World Aids Day fell on December 1st, as always and Jianbuo invited me and the Professor to spend the day with him in Dali to help distribute leaflets and talk to local people. When this special day arrived, we were met by an almost carnival-like atmosphere, a beautiful warm sunny day and a smiling Jianbuo. There were red balloons and glittery decorations around his stand in the centre of town where Chinese pop music emanated from a pair of loud speakers which had been placed nearby. Hundreds and hundreds of red ribbon emblems sat on scarlet cloth-covered tables next to information leaflets. Piles of little red and gold coloured packages containing information leaflets and condoms were placed nearby. Groups of young singing and dancing girls, and local acrobatic teams had been organised to entertain the crowds at intervals throughout the day, as were local musicians. This amiable, popular young man had produced colourful posters advertising the event, and was receiving full support from both his senior doctors at the Dali Number Two Hospital, and the team from the Anti-epidemic centre. I spent an enjoyable day with him handing out leaflets and pinning Red Ribbon emblems on shirts and blouses and enjoying the company. That evening I was tired but happy, knowing that we had had a successful day with all expenses covered by the very last of our monetary donation.

Every penny of the brilliant contribution from The Global Issues Command, facilitated by Simon Johnson at the British

Embassy and supported by VSO, had been spent on the much-needed cause to educate and spread awareness of HIV to the many people in the Dali Prefecture. I hadn't worked alone, and without the constant help and support of Martin Gordon of the Barry and Martin's Trust, who sponsored not only me, but also many of our early training sessions, VSO and the local NGOs situated in Kunming, we would not have been able to achieve any level of success. What an amazing journey I'd experienced.

My last few weeks at the college were hectic. I went to Dali and had lunch in my favourite eatery; Jacks Café, with Jack, Stella, Jianbuo and Langer. We chatted and reminisced for hours and hours and I didn't want to leave.

An evening was spent with the English teachers who Rumei had introduced me to on my arrival. These people had opened their homes to me and we spent many happy days together.

I went back to the Affiliated Hospital and spent time with Yang Kaishun, the doctor who fixed my ankle. His wife and little girl had joined him and he was a happy man. I felt sad when I said goodbye as this thoughtful man had helped me in more ways than one when I first arrived at his non-functioning hospital.

I spent a day with the Chen family who had lived in the flat above me, nearly three years earlier. They'd never forgotten me when I moved to the Medical College and frequently invited me to their home. I would certainly miss my five a side football matches with Chen Wen Jia and his friends.

I shared my special final moments in China with the delightful Rumei, her daughter Xinran and her charming parents who never failed to welcome me into their home. Without such a competent and willing interpreter, I would have achieved little or nothing, and I have a lot to thank her for. I felt sad as I was preparing to leave and hoped to see all these people, and those I haven't mentioned, again one day. I knew I would miss them.

During my taxi ride to the airport in Dali I reminisced over the three years that I had spent in Yunnan in the Peoples Republic of China: the loneliness and depression I had endured in the early days of living in this strange country, the gradual understanding of a different culture, getting to know its people and gaining trust, had at times been more difficult than I could ever possibly imagine. I had witnessed hardship caused by poverty, discrimination, and ignorance, and wept over conditions that hopefully would improve in the future. As my spirits lifted, I knew that through me, many lives would be saved. Those carrying and suffering from HIV or AIDS would now be treated with a better understanding from their families, friends and carers. I had done my best. These memories will remain with me forever. I checked in. The plane was waiting on the tarmac. I was going home.

The Peggy Health Centre.

Dr Zhang Jianbuo continued the work in caring for individuals with HIV and AIDS when I left. This was at a time when there was still a great reluctance from the authorities to accept the situation. However, things began to change in 2002 and he was able to start his project within the confines of the Dali Number Two Peoples' Hospital with the encouragement of a new leader.

In 2004 a new building was constructed in true Bai architectural style in the grounds of the old missionary hospital. The old Chapel and bell tower remain standing. The centre has a backdrop of the beautiful Cangshan Mountains and was funded by the Barry and Martin's Trust and the local municipality. This facility includes rooms for counselling, inpatients, outpatients, numerous clinics and is run by Dr Zhang Jianbuo.

I was present at the inauguration and felt both humbled and honoured when it was named the Peggy Health Centre.

This AIDS unit is quoted as not only being unique in China, but is also regarded nationally as one of the best units in the country and is held as an example to others. Through my recognition of a need, my work contributed greatly towards the creation of this clinic, and I am proud to be included in this legacy to the people of Dali and the surrounding area.

Acknowledgments

Thank you to Martin Gordon OBE, Chairman of Barry and Martin's Trust for sponsoring much of my time with Voluntary Services Overseas. This allowed me, together with my Chinese Medical colleagues at Dali Medical College, to recognise and provide the much-needed HIV awareness and crucial education programme to so many people throughout the Dali Prefecture.

Your support during my time in China was invaluable. Through your Trust you funded two HIV experts, Penny and Fiona from the Chelsea and Westminster Hospital, to visit us way down in a corner of south west China. They shared their knowledge and expertise with senior medical and nursing personnel at a conference in Kunming, the capital city of the Yunnan Province. From that first seminar, my confidence soared and my role escalated beyond belief.

Your Trust is recognised in many parts of the Peoples' Republic of China and your efforts to promote HIV and AIDS education, prevention, treatment and care to all, grows annually.

I feel honoured to know you Martin, and value our friendship.

Thank you, Simon Johnson for visiting us at the Medical College in Dali. Your keen interest in our proposed venture, and the subsequent financial aid you were able to facilitate, made the whole project viable. I was, and still am, very grateful Simon. Thank you.

Thank you to Voluntary Services Overseas for accepting me as a volunteer, thus providing me with the unforgettable experience of spending time in such a beautiful part of China with such interesting and delightful people. Sometimes life was tough, but mostly I was happy and know a little part of my heart will remain in Dali forever.

A special thank you to Zhang Rumei, my Chinese interpreter, who cared so much and became my friend during my stay when I was so far away from my home and family. Thank you so much Rumei for everything, you are often in my thoughts.

Finally, I would like to thank the Paphos Writers Group, Marian Taylor, Pamela Holland, Carole Manuel and Sara Dunn for encouraging me to get my story down on paper!

Lightning Source UK Ltd.
Milton Keynes UK
'KHW02f1544231117
13216UK00007B/256/P